Spiralizer Recipe Book

Recipes for weight loss

Author

Cathy M. Liston

Contents

CHAPTER 1

SPIRALIZING TOOLS

Using the right tool for the job is—as any handyman/woman knows—the key to success; you don't use a hammer to tighten a screw. There are three kinds of vegetable slicers on the market, and all have strengths and weaknesses you should be aware of when making a choice. (Or buy all three and have options!)

The Veggetti Spiral Vegetable Slicer

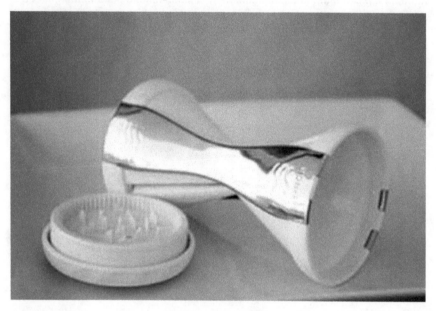

Best for: quick set up, small quantities of noodles, small "footprint" on the counter, and traveling.

This inventive, hourglass-shaped kitchen utensil is easy to use, easy to clean, and lightweight enough to carry with you when you travel. If you can imagine a pencil sharpener large enough to accommodate a zucchini, then you've just imagined the Veggetti Spiral Vegetable Slicer and how it works.

As with anything in your kitchen that has a blade—blender, food processor, silverware drawer—the Veggetti can bite if you're not careful. The blades are extremely sharp, so you need to be alert while you're turning your vegetables into delicious, low-calorie spaghetti strands. Most mishaps occur when a hand slips while guiding the vegetable through the blades, or when someone sticks a finger into the blade during cleaning.

Keep in mind that very little force is necessary. All you need to do is gently twist your vegetables through, preferably using the Veggetti's cap to grip the vegetable while you're twisting it.

Here's how to use the Veggetti safely:

STEP 1: Leave the skin on the gripping end of the vegetable. This gives you a more solid and less slippery surface to grip while you're twisting the vegetable into the Veggetti.

Notes: For most vegetables—such as zucchinis, carrots, yellow squash—I simply grip the end of the vegetable with my hand. However, the Veggetti comes with a "cap" that has little spikes which help to grip slippery vegetables. I find that this cap works well for dense vegetables (carrots), but not for soft vegetables (zucchini). In my experience, the cap will shred the end of soft vegetables, making it even more difficult to push them through the Veggetti. Another option to get the last inch of goodness out of each vegetable, is to stab a fork into the vegetable instead of using your fingers or the cap.

STEP 2: the Veggetti cutter looks like an hourglass with two open ends. Each "funnel" has a different blade so that you can vary the type of vegetable pasta you get—spaghetti-type strands or wider, udon noodles. Choose the width of noodle you want and guide your vegetable into that blade.

Notes: You'll quickly develop a preference for either the spaghetti or the udon noodle size for each vegetable. I love both, depending on the dish. Generally, I prefer the thinner spaghetti noodles for denser vegetables (carrots, beets, etc). For raw or lightly cooked dishes, I also prefer the thinner spaghetti noodles. However, the thicker udon noodles are great for soups, or dishes with thick sauces.

STEP 3: Once your vegetable is cleaned, scrubbed, or peeled, simply place the end you want to cut into the Veggetti and begin turning it, just as you would when sharpening a pencil. The "pasta" strands will begin appearing as soon as the turning starts. Discard the left over portion of the vegetable or save it for another use, like enriching soup.

Notes: Keep your fingers away from the blades! The Veggetti is known to bite if you're not careful. The best way to keep your fingers safe is to make sure the part of the vegetable you're gripping is dry, unpeeled, and firm. Otherwise use the Veggetti's cap or use a fork to grip the vegetable while you're spiralizing it.

For zucchini, I like to leave the stem on and use it as a grip while spiralizing. I find this to work so well that I never use the Veggetti's cap or a fork when spiralizing zucchini.

For carrots, parsnips, yellow squash, and other vegetables shaped like cones, I like to hold the thin end while spiralizing the thick end so I can use more and waste less of the vegetable.

For eggplant, I like to use the thicker cut because the thinner pasta strands are more fragile than the thicker pasta. Keep in mind that eggplant noodles are notoriously fragile and break easily.

One trick I've learned is to hold the Veggetti a little differently than shown in the manufacturer's instructions. The spiralizing process tends to produce a lot of excess "vegetable" matter and it can get a little messy, with bits of veggie goop falling out the opposite end of the Veggetti and into your plate. I like to cup that end of the Veggetti with my left hand when I spiralize with my right hand. This allows me to catch the vegetable goop in my palm so I can discard it easily.

The Veggetti works best with vegetables that have a tubular shape like zucchini, or cone-like shape like a carrot. The vegetable needs to be able to fit into the blades, and you need to be able to turn the vegetable easily in order to produce nice pasta strands. Therefore, any irregular shaped vegetable, or any oversized or undersized vegetable will not work very well. Use this tool for vegetables sized between 1-1/2" and 2-1/2" diameter. Anything smaller causes too much waste, and anything larger simply cannot fit!

- Zucchini—snip the nose off the zucchini, and use the stem on the other end as a handle to guide the vegetable through the cutter.
- Yellow squash—snip the nose off the squash, and hold the vegetable along the thin end (the stem end) so that the thicker part of the vegetable is turned into noodles and there's less waste.
- Cucumbers—snip the nose off, peel most of the skin but make sure to leave the skin on the gripping end so your hand doesn't slip!
- Carrots, Turnips, and other similar roots—cut ½" from the stem end (the thick end) and grip the thin end. This provides more noodle and less waste. Be careful to choose carrots that are not cracked, as cracks will cause short circles instead of long strands of pasta.
- Sweet Potatoes, Yams, Potatoes, Beets—if the potato or beet is large, you may need to cut it down to a size that can be handled by the Veggetti. Be VERY careful with these vegetables, they are slippery and can easily cause injury. I always use the Veggetti cap to grip these vegetables while spiralizing.

Worst veggies to use with the Veggetti:
- Apples—too large and too difficult to grip.
- Eggplants—too large, and the pasta strands can easily fall apart.
- Vegetables with irregular shapes.

The Paderno Spiralizer

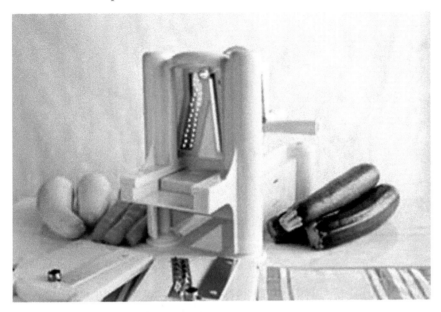

Best for: large quantities of noodles, and greater variety of cuts and shreds. It takes more counter space and more time to set up than a Veggetti, but once it's set up, it works much faster

The Paderno Spiralizer is a hand-powered tool, which means it is neither battery-powered nor electrical. About the size of a counter-top mixer, it is safer than other hand-held vegetable spiralizers, such as the Veggetti, because the vegetable is inserted into the machine, and directed toward the cutting blades by the action of a turning crank—the cook's hands never get anywhere near the sharp surfaces.

The Paderno has three blades that produce three different types of noodles:

Thin Spaghetti-sized noodles

Thick udon/linguini-size noodles

Wide, flat lasagna noodles—the width depending on the diameter of the vegetable/fruit being cut. This blade also shreds certain vegetables like cabbage, which makes it useful for quickly making slaws and salads.

Here's how to use the Paderno safely:

STEP 1: Make certain the machine is firmly "seated" on the counter and that all four suction cups are "engaged." You do this by simply pushing down on the Paderno's legs. Put your body into it! If you don't set the suction cups, as soon as you start using the machine, it will slide right off the counter. To release the suction, simply break the seal by pushing a finger under the suction cups.

STEP 2: Select the appropriate blade depending on how you want to process your vegetable. There are three blades provided with this slicer (thin, thick, and wide).

STEP 3: Sandwich the vegetable to be spiralized or shredded into the machine, holding it in place with the prongs. Be careful to center the vegetable against the blade as well as you can, otherwise it will be more difficult to spiralize.

STEP 4: With your left hand, push the lever forward toward the blade, while turning the crank with your right hand to cut the vegetable. Keep firm pressure against the blade to produce the best results. Do not push on the crank as that might break it. To get shorter "pasta" pieces, cut a groove in the vegetable so that when the "spirals" are sliced off, they are automatically cut, creating the smaller (short) pasta shapes.

Notes: I've found that dense vegetables (such as beets and jicama) can be difficult to successfully spiralize. The Paderno's blades don't always cut deeply enough to slice all the way through, producing full-width noodles that look scored instead of cut. The reason is because dense vegetables require more force to keep them lined up correctly on the blades. But applying too much force to the Paderno can break it. Unfortunately, I haven't found a reliable way to handle this problem other than to grip the lever closer to its hinge and apply more pressure while turning the crank very carefully.

Quirks: Some vegetables may need to be trimmed a bit so that it will easily fit into the center blade.

With some vegetables you'll need to cut a bit off the vegetable so that the crank end will grip it properly. Simply slice off a piece to flatten the end of the vegetable and push the flat end into the prongs to secure it. (With apples, you don't need to do anything except stick the fruit on the crank and start turning.)

Best veggies to use with the Paderno Spiralizer:

The Paderno is particularly good with soft and less dense vegetables and can easily handle larger vegetables that have a diameter of up to 5 inches.

- Apples—particularly nice when cut into the "udon" size
- Cabbages—great for shredding.
- Zucchini—terrific for large zucchini.
- Yellow Squash—also terrific if the squash is large enough.
- Onions—for fast shredding.
- Larger vegetables (up to 5 inches in diameter)

Worst veggies to use with the Paderno spiralizer

- Beets—are difficult for the Paderno to slice because they are so dense and tough. Turn the crank slowly for best results. And always peel the beet before spiralizing.
- Carrots, Turnips, etc—unless you can find huge carrots or turnips, most carrots are simply too small in diameter to be spiralized by the Paderno. Large carrots also have a tendency to crack on the Paderno. Use a Veggetti or Julienne slicer instead.
- Small zucchini—if your zucchini is less than 1-1/2" in diameter, it will produce more waste than noodles in the Paderno. Use a Veggetti or Julienne slicer instead.

The Julienne Slicer and Mandoline

Best for: precision slicing, matchstick cuts, difficult vegetables and fruit, portability.

This is the 21st century version of the cooking tool first known as the "mandoline." It is a low-tech tool with no moving parts, just a set of wicked sharp blades that create different sizes and styles of vegetable slices, including crinkle-cut vegetables for "fries."

Best for: nice flat "lasagna" ribbons ranging from thick to ultra-thin, and julienne-cut vegetables

While it is a low-tech gadget, it has been maximized to make it easy to adjust thicknesses while slicing allowing for cuts from paper-thin to thick. There is a purpose-built julienne blade included that will allow for perfect "matchstick" cuts as well. Although the spiralizer-style cutters can create julienne strips, the mandoline is a fast alternative to chopping by hand and is also easier to clean than either the Veggetti or the Paderno style spiralizers.

Best veggies to use with a Mandoline / Julienne Slicer: any!

How To Clean Your Spiralizer

The number one easiest way to clean each of these wonderful spiralizing tools is to wash them under running water immediately after use. If you wash immediately after using, then any vegetable matter will easily slough off of the tool and its blades. Warm soapy water is more effective as it softens the vegetable matter even more. Simply run water over the blades, and use your kitchen brush if needed, then put the tool on your drying rack. The entire process takes 30 seconds.

If you don't clean your spiralizer right away, then you'll have some extra work to do. The entire Veggetti is dishwasher-proof, as are the blades on the Paderno, so for the most part, all you need to do is throw the appliance in the dishwasher and hit "go." But there are times when particles of vegetable matter will cling to the blades. When that happens, there are two easy ways to clean out the debris without putting your fingers at risk.

One method is to use hot water with the sink power sprayer to force the particles out. The second is to use a clean toothbrush to gently scrub the sharp surfaces. (Buy them by the handful at the dollar store and keep a couple in your utensil drawer. You'll be amazed at how useful they'll be.)

For Julienne slicers of any type, hand-washing is recommended. Use the power-rinse at your sink and run hot water through the device to remove any food debris. Wash immediately after use if cutting zucchini or beets, which can leave stains.

CHAPTER 2

ALL ABOUT VEGETABLES

Not all vegetables and fruits work with each type of cutter. Each different type of vegetable cutter has its pros, cons, and quirks. For example, a tomato can be sliced by a mandolin-type slicer, but it would turn to mush in a Veggetti or Paderno-style spiralizer. Nor can you spiralize vegetables and fruits with pits (avocados, stone fruits).

You can't spiralize vegetables that are smaller than 1 ½ inches in diameter. That category would include asparagus, green beans, and Chinese long beans. Very soft ingredients—like bananas—also don't work well in a spiralizer-type cutter, and neither will fruits like kiwi and watermelon that are mostly water. But again, the mandolin-style slicers work fine for these vegetables or fruits.

What Are The Best Vegetables (and Fruits) To Spiralize?

Here is a list of vegetables and fruits which I've found to spiralize well:

Apples

Nutrition: Apples are nutrient filled and fiber rich. A medium apple has approximately 115 calories and a low glycemic index (GI) number of 37.

They also provide, among other vitamins and minerals, 28% of the RDA of vitamin C.

Best way to spiralize: Apples range from tart to super sweet and any of the three basic kinds of vegetable cutter will work well with them. For best results, use firm apples without any soft spots. Leave the peel on to add a bit of color to the noodles.

Cooking tips: best eaten raw or baked.

Beets

Nutrition: These low-calorie, high-fiber and zero cholesterol roots contain antioxidant vitamins A and C, which help protect against cardiovascular disease and reduce the risk of stroke. They also contain minerals such as iron, potassium, copper, magnesium, and manganese—all of which are important in maintaining optimum health of systems.

Best way to spiralize: Beets are dense, hard vegetables and can be difficult to spiralize with a Paderno. I recommend using either a Julienne slicer or a Veggetti cutter. You may need to cut the beet down to less than 2-1/2" diameter, and slightly shape it with a knife before spiralizing it with the Veggetti.

Cooking tips: Beets can be eaten raw, or cooked. Let the recipe or your own inspiration guide you.

Bell peppers

Nutrition: Bell peppers of any color are rich sources of vitamin C and carotenoids, powerful antioxidants that have been shown to significantly reduce the likelihood of lung cancer.

Best way to spiralize: They work best with the mandoline-type slicers, whose precise cuts make for a professional presentation in dishes as diverse as sukiyaki and salads.

Cooking tips: They can be eaten raw or cooked.

Broccoli

Nutrition: Broccoli is one of the cancer-fighting cruciferous vegetables, and contains more vitamin C than an orange.

Best way to spiralize: The fibrous stalks are difficult to slice in either a Veggetti or Paderno— they're too irregularly shaped for the Veggetti and they split on the Paderno. However, the mandolin-style cutters will provide neat julienne slices faster and more uniformly than using a chef's knife will.

Cooking tips: The fibrous stalks of broccoli are perfect for short veggie pasta but they should be blanched before eating to cut down on the strong taste.

Cabbage

Nutrition: Like broccoli, cabbage belongs to the cruciferous vegetable family. (Other members include Brussels sprouts, bok choy, and cresses. All varieties of cabbage contain sinigrin, an anti-cancer nutrient but Savoy cabbage is a particularly good source.

Best way to spiralize: Cabbage cannot be cut into pasta strands, but it shreds very well on the Paderno. You can vary the size of the shreds by choosing different Paderno blades. If using a Paderno slicer to shred cabbage for slaws or stir-fries, it's best to use a small head.

Cooking tips: It can be eaten raw, but steaming the vegetable makes it particularly effective for lowering cholesterol.

Cauliflower

Nutrition: Cauliflower is nutritionally dense—low in carbohydrates but high in fiber, folate (necessary for nerve health and emotional well-being), and antioxidant vitamin C. It is also high in vitamin K, which is essential for effective blood clotting. Cauliflower contains phytochemicals which have been shown to protect against various kinds of cancer.

Best way to spiralize: The "wide" blade of the Paderno slicer is perfect for turning cauliflower into "rice" or "couscous." If a finer grain is desired, you can also process it further in a food processor.

Cooking tips: Cauliflower should be cooked before eating. Because the texture of cauliflower rice is important, I recommend following the recipe's cooking instructions.

Carrots

Nutrition: A medium sized carrot has only 52 calories, 12 grams of carbohydrate, 4 grams of fiber and is one of the best natural sources of vitamin A. Carrots also contain iron, B6 and other B vitamins, manganese, vitamins E, K and C, along with phosphorus, choline, potassium and calcium. Carrots are naturally sweet.

Best way to spiralize: Carrots are often a little small for the Paderno, so they are best spiralized in a Veggetti cutter, or a mandoline-style slicer for uniform julienne cuts.

Cooking tips: Eat them raw (thin carrot noodles are delicious raw), warm them with sauce or in soup, or cook them briefly in boiling water.

Celeriac

Nutrition: Touted as an underrated vegetable by Epicurious and Martha Stewart, Celeriac is also known as "celery root." This root vegetable looks like a turnip and tastes much like the better known vegetable "celery." Unlike most other root vegetables, celeriac contains almost no starch. The vegetable contains large amounts of vitamin K (important for blood clotting), as well as C and B vitamins.

Best way to spiralize: It works well in all three types of vegetable slicers.

Cooking tips: It can be eaten raw or cooked, and is often mashed as a substitute for potatoes on weight-loss diets.

Chayote Squash

Nutrition: Chayote squash generally look like big green pears. It is high in potassium and low in sodium.

Best way to spiralize: All three slices can be used on this vegetable, but it has to be cut into smaller pieces for the Veggetti.

Cooking tips: It can be eaten raw or cooked and its extremely mild flavor makes it perfect for pasta dishes where a more assertively flavored noodle (like broccoli) would overpower the taste.

Citrus Fruit (only for the mandolin-type slicer)

All you'll get is pulpy juice if you try to spiralize citrus fruit with a Paderno or Veggetti slicer. But a mandolin-style slicer is the perfect tool for shaving precise slices on everything from a tiny kumquat to a ruby red grapefruit. Whether the slices are being used as an essential ingredient—in something like a tomato quiche or a pitcher of sangria—or a garnish for a platter of poached salmon, the citrus fruit adds more than a spark of taste,

Cucumber

Nutrition: Cucumbers are related to the squash family and contain high amounts of vitamin K as well as antioxidant and anti-inflammatory substances. They are most often enjoyed as an ingredient in soups or salads.

Best way to spiralize: They work well with all spiralizers slicers. The Veggetti and Paderno produce easy noodles, while the mandoline-style slicers produce lovely cucumber salad slices.

Cooking tips: Cucumbers can be eaten raw or cooked, peeled or intact.

Eggplant

Nutrition: Eggplant contains important phytonutrients and antioxidants like nasunin, which protects the circulatory system.

Best way to spiralize: Eggplant is difficult to spiralize with a Veggetti, but the wide, flat eggplant "lasagna noodles' made with a Paderno slicer or a mandoline slicer make an excellent base for traditional recipes like moussaka and lasagna.

Cooking tips: Eggplant should not be eaten raw. Roasting is particularly delicious way of cooking eggplant. Some recipes are better if you salt the raw eggplant and let the water drain out prior to cooking.

Jerusalem artichoke

Nutrition: Also known as "sunchoke" or "sunroot," the Jerusalem artichoke is actually a species of sunflower. It is often used as a substitute for potatoes because of its satisfyingly starchy texture. It is a rich source of the B vitamin thiamine, providing 20 percent of the RDA.

Best way to spiralize: Because of its size, it works well with the Paderno and mandoline-style slicers.

Cooking tips: They can be eaten raw but may cause "gas" if eaten in that state.

Jicama

Nutrition: Also known as "yambean," jicama is a rich source of the antioxidant vitamin C and nerve-protecting B vitamins as well as several trace minerals including potassium, which protects against heart disease. Other nutrients found in jicama are anti-inflammatory and anti-viral.

Best way to spiralize: Jicama is too large to spiralize in a Veggetti unless you cut it down to manageable size. It is also quite dense, which requires extra care to spiralize in a Paderno. A Julienne slicer works particularly well with jicama.

Cooking tips: It can be eaten raw and is often sold as a street snack in Mexico, sprinkled with lime juice and chili powder.

Leeks

Nutrition: Leeks are an extremely healthy food, with almost 30% of the RDA for vitamin K as well as 13% of the RDA for manganese, which is important for reproductive health.

Best way to spiralize: Leeks make lovely ribbons of flat pasta that work well in soups, salads, and pasta dishes. They can be spiralized, Paderno-ized, and sliced with a mandoline.

Cooking tips: Like other members of the allium family, leeks can be eaten raw, but the are best when cooked to al dente perfection. My favorite way of serving any size or shape of leek is blanched with a sprinkle of olive oil and French sea salt.

Onion

Nutrition: Onions are a member of the "allium family," along with garlic, shallots, and leeks, and like its fellow family members, it is rich in flavonoids, including quercetin, which has antioxidant and anti-inflammatory properties that protect the circulatory system and male reproductive system.

Best way to spiralize: The Paderno slicer shreds onions in seconds with no tears, but mandoline-style slicers are also useful for cutting uniform slices. (Onion rings anyone?)

Parsnip

Nutrition: Parsnips are a surprisingly sweet root vegetable and contain almost as much sugar as the average banana. In addition to anti-inflammatory, anti-fungal, and anti-cancer properties, parsnips are good sources of folate, vitamin C, and vitamins K and E.

Best way to spiralize: Like carrots, parsnips work best in the Veggetti or mandoline-style cutters unless they're very large (over two inches in diameter), in which case a Paderno works brilliantly.

Cooking tips: Baking and roasting are my preferred ways to cook Parsnips.

Pear

Slicing up a pears for desserts like clafouti or pie is a lot faster using either the Veggetti or Paderno slicer. There's no need to peel the fruit, simply wash and dry well before beginning the slicing process. (Pear skins have three to four times the nutrient value of the rest of the fruit, and those nutrients include antioxidants, anti-inflammatory and anti-cancer substances.) Extra bonus for diabetics—the flavonoids in pears can improve insulin sensitivity.

Plantain

Nutrition: Green plantains are starchy but low in sugar (as long as you don't fry them). Plantains are good sources of copper, manganese, potassium, and magnesium, as well as vitamins A and B-6, which protects against stroke and other cardiovascular events. For best results use the straightest and firmest plantains you can find.

Best way to spiralize: Unlike their botanical cousins bananas, plantains are firm enough to stand up to any kind of veggie cutter.

Cooking tips: Plantains need to be cooked before eating. They can be pan-fried, grilled and baked.

Potatoes

Nutrition: While potatoes have a bad rep, a medium-sized potato only contains about 100 calories while delivering significant amounts of the antioxidant vitamins A and C, B6 and other B vitamins, as well as bone-building calcium and magnesium, potassium, and phosphorus.

Best way to spiralize: If the potato is small enough, both thin and thick blades on a Veggetti spiralizer works well. For large potatoes or large quantities, use a Paderno and choose the blade that best fits the recipe.

Cooking tips: Always cook potatoes before eating. Potato noodles can fall apart when boiled.

Pumpkin

Nutrition: Pumpkin can be substituted for any other type of squash. Pumpkin noodles are mildly flavored and colorful. Pumpkin "fries" are a low-calorie, low cholesterol, and low sodium substitute for traditional fries and they deliver hefty doses of vitamins A, C, and E, as well as B vitamins, including folic acid, and potassium, copper, and manganese.

Best way to spiralize: Pumpkin needs to be cut down before it can be spiralized. As long as you cut the pumpkin to a somewhat regular shape, it can be spiralized by a Veggetti or Paderno. However, because of the extra effort involved in cutting pumpkin to an appropriate shape for spiralizing, I prefer to use a julienne slicer for quick pumpkin noodles or matchsticks.

Cooking tips: Baking and roasting are preferred ways to cook pumpkin noodles, but check the recipe for specifics.

Radishes

Nutrition: Radishes are low-carb, low-calorie cancer fighters filled with immune-boosting vitamin C as well as vitamin K and B complex vitamins. Their mineral content (potassium, calcium, manganese, iron, phosphorus, zinc, and copper) help promote healthy bones and support optimum health.

Best way to spiralize: Because radishes are so small, they're difficult to spiralize with either Veggetti or Paderno slicers. However a julienne slicer can easily produce beautifully thin slices or matchsticks.

Cooking tips: Radishes are excellent raw.

Squash

Nutrition: All varieties of squash are low-calorie, low-carb, cholesterol-free, and high in fiber. They are also high in the antioxidant vitamins A and C, and contain significant amounts of niacin, folic acid, potassium, and iron. Squashes are anti-inflammatory and contain no fat.

Best way to spiralize: Yellow squash is very easy to spiralize with either Veggetti, Paderno or julienne slicers. Other squashes can require cutting with a knife prior to spiralizing. My strong preference is to use yellow squash when possible, as the results are consistently wonderful with this commonly available squash.

Cooking tips: If it is fresh, yellow squash is sweet and delicious raw. However, it quickly develops a bitter taste when it is no longer fresh. Cook yellow squash lightly, or it will turn mushy and lose its wonderful texture and flavor. My preferred way to prepare squash is blanched with a little olive oil and sea salt.

Sweet Potato

Nutrition: The sweet potato is rich in antioxidants like beta-carotene and has a lower glycemic index (70) compared to a white potato (111).

Best way to spiralize: Sweet potatoes are hard, dense vegetables that can be difficult to spiralize. If less than 2-1/2" in diameter, try spiralizing with a Veggetti. Make sure to peel the part you want to spiralize, and leave the peel on the part you're holding. For a Paderno, peel it and cut both ends, and carefully spiralize with either blade. Sweet potatoes make excellent noodles and julienne-sliced "fries."

Cooking tips: Sweet potatoes should not be eaten raw. Boiling the noodles too long can cause them to fall apart.

Tomatoes

You can't spiralize tomatoes but you can use a handheld mandoline like the Microplane to slice them paper thin. Tomatoes can be eaten raw or cooked. Tomatoes are botanically fruit and their juicy flesh is a rich source of lycopene, a nutrient that can—among other things—limit and repair sun damage on skin.

Turnip

Nutrition: Turnips are an excellent source of anti-oxidants, minerals, vitamins and dietary fiber. They provide a healthy dose of vitamin C while containing only 28 calories per 100g.

Best way to spiralize: Like beets and rutabaga, turnips are hard and dense, which makes them difficult to spiralize. Try spiralizing in a Veggetti, taking care not to slip and cut your fingers. If the turnip is large enough, a Paderno may be used. As with the other dense vegetables, a julienne slicer may be a better tool to use.

Yam

Nutrition: Vitamin-rich yams are often mistaken for sweet potatoes but they are in fact, a completely different species of plant, a relative to flowers and grasses native to North Africa.

Best way to spiralize: They are large, dense vegetables and may be difficult for the Paderno to process. The Veggetti can spiralize them easily if the vegetable is cut into slices that will fit into the cutter. A julienne slicer can also work well.

Cooking tips: Yams should be peeled and cooked before eating as they contain toxins.

Zucchini

Nutrition: Zucchini is so popular as a vegetable alternative to wheat and rice pasta that it the green noodles are now called "zoodles." Zucchini is high in the antioxidant vitamins A and C, as well as Folate (critical for nerve health) and other B vitamins, as well as vitamin K. Low in sodium and cholesterol, Zucchini is a low-calorie source of dietary fiber and the minerals Phosphorus, Copper, Magnesium, Potassium, and Manganese.

Best way to spiralize: Zucchinis work very well with the Veggetti and mandoline-style slicers. If using the Paderno, choose fat, straight zucchini for best results.

Cooking tips: Fresh zucchini can be eaten raw, peeled or unpeeled. Often, if the recipe is a hot dish, simply mixing the raw zucchini noodles with the hot ingredients will "cook" the zucchini noodles enough to be perfectly and enjoyably "al dente." If you prefer your zucchini noodles to be cooked longer, then I recommend blanching for a few minutes and removing the cooked noodles from the pot to prevent overcooking.

How To Prepare and Cook Your Vegetable "Pasta"

Cooking your vegetable pasta is even easier than cooking traditional pasta! Here's how:

RAW

Most of the pasta you make from fruits and vegetables can be eaten raw. The exceptions are potatoes, sweet potatoes, and eggplant. Raw sweet potato contains an enzyme inhibitor that blocks the digestion of protein. Raw potatoes absorb bacteria from the soil and water (listeria, E. coli, and salmonella). They should be cooked before eating to destroy the bacteria. Raw eggplant contains a substance that inhibits the absorption of calcium and can also cause neurological and digestive problems.

Note: For most thin noodles made with soft vegetables (zucchini, yellow squash), mixing the warm or piping hot sauce with the raw noodles "cooks" them to just the desired "al dente" firmness.

WARMED

Warm the pasta strands by microwaving them for a few seconds in a microwave-safe bowl or by quickly "blanching" them in hot water before serving. (To blanch, bring a large pot of water to a boil. When the water is boiling, drop the noodles in and continue to heat for anywhere from 30 seconds to 10 minutes, depending on the vegetable. (Soft vegetables like zucchini or yellow squash take about 30 seconds; carrots take several minutes, beets can take as long as 10 minutes.)

BOILED

You will not need to "boil" your vegetable pasta unless you like the texture soft, bordering on mushy. Some vegetable pasta--white potatoes for instance--will simply fall apart after being boiled. An alternative cooking method would be "steaming," where the vegetable pasta is put in a wire steaming basket and cooked over boiling water without actually being immersed in it.

TIP: if you undercook the pasta just a little, then drizzle with virgin olive oil, you'll never want to cook it any other way.

SAUTÉED

This is a simple technique for cooking the pasta and other ingredients quickly. The ingredients are placed in a pan—either a saucepan or a skillet—with a little fat or oil and cooked over high heat. The trick with this method is to stir often to prevent the ingredients from burning.

STIR-FRIED

Stir-frying is a quick-cooking method that requires very little fat. The secret to successful stir-fries is pre-prep. All the ingredients should be chopped or cut as needed so that everything will cook quickly. Woks are purpose-built for stir-frying, but any large, heavy skillet will do as well.

Here's a quick primer on how to stir fry:

- Make sure your ingredients are dry.
- Heat the oil over high heat, then add the aromatic ingredients (garlic, chilis, onions) and spices to the oil before adding any other ingredients. This allows the flavors to infuse the oil.
- Add the rest of the ingredients, being careful not to overcrowd the pan. If necessary cook in small batches.
- As with sautéing, you need to pay attention to the process; stir-frying is done over high heat and the ingredients can easily burn.

BAKED

Pasta in traditional dishes like mac and cheese has to be boiled first before being combined with the cheese sauce and baked. With vegetable noodles, you can simply add the raw noodles to the ingredients—they'll cook while the dish is baking, thus saving you a step. Keep in mind that vegetable noodles cook much more quickly than wheat pasta, therefore your baking times will be considerably shorter than usual.

How Much "Pasta" Will It Make?

For most traditional pasta recipes, the default ingredient is 1 pound of pasta, which yields 4 cups of cooked pasta. In the following recipes, 4 cups of vegetable spaghetti will be the standard ingredient. To get 4 cups of vegetable pasta from your veggies use the following guide. Equivalents are approximate depending on the size of the vegetable.

- Beets — 8 medium beets, trimmed = 4 cups beat pasta
- Broccoli — 6-8 trimmed broccoli stalks = 4 cups broccoli pasta
- Carrot — 8 medium carrots = 4 cups carrot pasta
- Cauliflower — 1 head of trimmed cauliflower = 4 cups cauliflower "rice"
- Cucumbers — 3-4 medium cucumbers = 4 cups cucumber pasta
- Jicama — 2 whole jicamas = 4 cups jicama pasta.
- Potato — 6 medium potatoes = 4 cups potato pasta
- Radish — 2 Daikon radishes = 4 cups radish pasta
- Squash — 4-6 yellow squash = 4 cups squash pasta
- Sweet Potato — 3 medium sweet potatoes = 4 cups sweet potato pasta
- Zucchini — 3-4 whole zucchini = 4 cups zucchini pasta

How To Store Leftover Vegetable Pasta

Leftover veggie noodles must be refrigerated, preferably in a container (glass or plastic) with an air-tight seal in the coldest part of the fridge. If the noodles have been cooked, or mixed with other hot ingredients, you can store them for up to 2 days. If the noodles are raw, they should be used within 24 hours. If you want to prevent discoloration, squeeze a little lemon juice over the raw pasta before storing.

CHAPTER 3

INGREDIENTS, TERMS & DIETS

"You don't have to cook fancy or complicated masterpieces - just good food from fresh ingredients."

— Julia Child

Recipe Tags

The recipes in this book are based on fresh veggie pastas made with common spiralizer and julienne veggie cutters available on the market today.

The recipes that follow are tagged:

Gluten-free Paleo Weight-Loss for Vegetarian Vegan

A Note On Ingredients

Unless otherwise noted, when a recipe calls for the following ingredients, you should use:

- Brown sugar—light brown sugar
- Butter—"sweet" (unsalted) butter
- Chicken, beef, or vegetable stock—low-sodium
- Olive oil—extra-virgin
- Salt—sea salt
- Soy sauce—low sodium, tamari-style
- Sugar—white, granulated
- Yogurt—unflavored, unsweetened, Greek-style

Prep Terms

Julienne—food cut into long, thin strips. "Shoestring fries" are julienned potatoes.

Matchstick—this is a thicker, more squared-off cut than a julienne and can range from thin (1/16th of an inch) to a 1/3 inch cut known in French as a batonnet cut.

Spiralized—this refers to vegetables or fruits cut into strands or spirals by using a Veggetti or Paderno slicer.

Rice or Couscous—refers to the small rice-like grains made by slicing Cauliflower head with a Veggetti or Paderno slicer. Try using the thick blade to make "rice" and the thin blade to make "couscous."

Pasta Terms

The spiralizer-type vegetable cutters used for this book create several different kinds of vegetable pasta, all of which are used in the recipes.

- Spaghetti (also interchangeable with Angel Hair)—refers to the long strands cut by the thin blades on either the Veggetti or the Paderno slicers.
- Udon (interchangeable with Linguini)—refers to the long strands cut by the thick blades on either the Veggetti or the Paderno slicers.
- Flat—refers to the long strands cut by the wide blade on the Paderno slicer, or the flat blade of a julienne slicer.
- Spaghetti Circles—the short, circular strands cut by scoring one side of a vegetable and slicing it with the thin blades on either the Veggetti or the Paderno slicers.
- Udon Circles—the short, circular strands cut by scoring one side of a vegetable and slicing it with the thick blades on either the Veggetti or the Paderno slicers.
- Flat Circles—the short, circular strands cut by scoring one side of a vegetable and slicing it the wide blade on the Paderno slicer.
- Spaghetti Semicircles—the short, semicircular strands cut by scoring both sides of a vegetable and slicing it with the thin blades on either the Veggetti or the Paderno slicers.
- Udon Semicircles—the short, semicircular strands cut by scoring both sides of a vegetable and slicing it with the thick blades on either the Veggetti or the Paderno slicers.
- Flat Semicircles—the short, semicircular strands cut by scoring both sides of a vegetable and slicing it the wide blade on the Paderno slicer.

Dietary Considerations

Gluten-Free (GF)

"Gluten "is the name given to several proteins found in cereal grains (wheat, barley, and rye are the biggest offenders, but it's also found in spelt and triticale, among other sources). Gluten makes dough more elastic, and is hidden in many foods under a variety of innocent-sounding ingredients. (For a full list of these gluten-containing ingredients, consult WebMD: http://www.webmd.com/diet/features/hidden-sources-of-gluten).

A growing body of research suggests that eating wheat — even in its whole form — contributes to a variety of health problems ranging from digestive disorders (Celiac disease, "leaky gut" syndrome) to obesity (what belly) and diabetes. There's even persuasive evidence that links wheat consumption to cognitive disorders ("grain brain").

Substituting fresh vegetable pasta for traditional wheat pasta is one small change that can result in huge benefits. Not only is eating "veggie pasta" a painless way to introduce more vegetables into any diet—always a good thing—but the increased fiber intake can help "reset" the body's metabolism, normalizing blood sugar, and replenishing depleted stocks of antioxidant vitamins and minerals, resulting in increased immune health.

For more information about gluten, contact The Celiac Disease Foundation http://celiac.org/live-gluten-free/glutenfreediet/what-is-gluten/

Glycemic Index (GI)

GI measures the impact a food has on the eater's blood sugar level. The scale basically ranges from 0-100, with 100 being the glycemic index of a slice of white bread. Diabetics and others with blood sugar issues are encouraged to eat low on the glycemic index, avoiding simple carbohydrates that metabolize into sugar quickly.

Glycemic Load (GL)

GL is a refinement of the measurement of glycemic index and takes into account the total makeup of a food, and not just its carbohydrates, as well as the portion size. Anything with a glycemic load under 10 is considered low glycemic. (Apples have a GL of 6; grapefruit is upper-low at 3.) A serving of Kraft macaroni and cheese comes in at a whopping GL of 32. Even adding in the milk and cheese to veggie noodle version, you'll still come out ahead, since the GL of a 4-oz. serving of zucchini is only 2.

Paleo

The Paleo Diet (aka "the Caveman Diet") is a back-to-basics food movement that focuses on the ingredients that were available to our caveman ancestors. That means no grains (cavemen were hunters, not farmers), no dairy and no sugar—the trifecta of ingredients responsible for the epidemic of obesity and the explosion of diabetes worldwide.

The Paleo diet also eliminates processed foods, including condiments like soy sauce, ketchup, and mustard, and all fats that are not plant-based. It's a very "clean" way of eating and ordinary pasta has no place on the Paleo plate. Veggie pasta, though, is wholeheartedly allowed.

Weight-Loss

Both Gluten-free and Paleo diets emphasize protein and "good carbs" and eliminate or limit sweets and grains. That's a good start for any weight-loss program. To lose weight you must do one of two things—eat less or exercise more, preferably both. But as any veteran dieter knows, not all calories are created equal. A cup of broccoli with humus will fill you up faster than a cup of chocolate pudding (which has triple the calories) will.

The recipes in this book are based on fresh veggie pastas made with the spiralizer and veggie cutters on the market today.

Salt

A special note about salt: the less the better, no matter what dietary plan you follow. A high-sodium intake stresses your kidneys, contributes to high blood-pressure, osteoporosis, diabetes, and water retention.

In general, all of the recipes in this book were created with an eye to lightening the sodium load. And really, any recipe that includes a high-salt ingredient like bacon, anchovies, or feta cheese really does not need additional salt. Try the recipes as is and you will be pleasantly surprised by how strongly flavored and delicious your food can be, even without a couple sprinkles of salt.

CHAPTER 4

SOUPS

Noodle soups are universally found throughout the world and are considered comfort food in any language. Starting a meal with a nutritious bowl of soup "takes the edge" off the appetite, and generally results in consuming less calories per meal, a boon for those watching their weight.

GF - Gluten-free   P - Paleo   WL - Weight-Loss   V - for Vegetarian   Vg - Vegan

thai chicken noodle soup (gf/p/wl)

This soup features three flavors that define Thai cuisine, coconut, chili, and lime.

Prep Time: 25–30 m

Serves: 4

Calories: 378, Sodium: 1208 mg, Dietary Fiber: 2.4 g, Total Fat: 21.6 g, Total Carbs: 17.0 g, Protein: 30.0 g

Ingredients

....

½ cup zucchini noodles, spaghetti cut

2 boneless, skinless chicken breasts cut into bite-size pieces

5 cups chicken broth

1 cup coconut milk (can use low-fat)

2 jalapeno peppers, seeded and chopped finely

2 large cloves garlic, chopped

1 ½ inch piece ginger root, grated

1 Tbsp. lime zest

¼ cup fresh lime juice

4 Tbsp. fish sauce (I use Red Boat)

2 cups shiitake mushrooms, sliced

2 cups baby spinach leaves

2 Tbsp. chopped cilantro

....

Method

- Combine the chicken broth, jalapeno, garlic, ginger, lime juice and zest and 3 Tbsp. fish sauce in a medium sauce pan and bring to a simmer.
- Add the noodles and cook for one minute or until tender. Use tongs to remove the noodles. Place in a bowl and cover to keep warm.
- Add the mushrooms to the simmering broth. Simmer for another four minutes, then add the chicken and the coconut milk.
- Continue to simmer until the chicken is cooked through.
- Add the spinach and stir until the leaves get limp, then add the chopped cilantro and remaining tablespoon of fish sauce.
- Divide the cooked noodles into four bowls and pour the soup over the noodles.

tunisian noodle soup (gf/p/wl)

This spicy noodle soup is a vegetarian African variation of the ubiquitous chicken noodle soup.

Prep Time: 25–30 m

Serves: 4–6

Calories: 181, Sodium: 184 mg, Dietary Fiber: 2.9 g, Total Fat: 10.0 g, Total Carbs: 20.7 g, Protein: 4.7 g

Ingredients

....

2 cups zucchini noodles, spaghetti cut

2 quarts vegetable stock (or chicken stock)

1 pound Swiss chard, chopped coarsely (stems, ribs, and eaves)

1 large red onion, chopped

3 large garlic cloves, minced

4 Tbsp. olive oil (or coconut oil)

2 Tbsp. tomato paste

2 Tbsp. hot pepper sauce

1 Tbsp. fresh lemon juice

....

Method

- Bring the stock to a boil in a stockpot. Add the chard and cook until the chard is wilted.
- Stir in the tomato paste, oil, hot pepper sauce, garlic, and onion. Return to a boil and then reduce to a simmer.
- Simmer for 5-10 minutes, then add the noodles. Cook for about 1 minute, or until they are tender.

mexican chicken noodle soup (gf/p/wl)

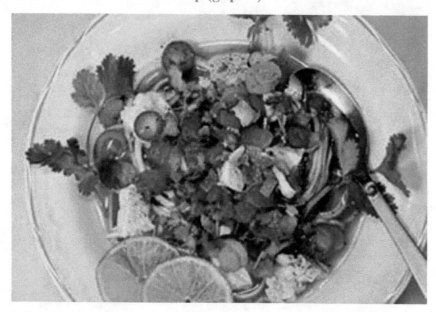

This spicy, tomato-based soup is another international variation of chicken noodle soup.

Prep Time: 25–30 m

Serves: 6

Calories: 592, Sodium: 1336 mg, Dietary Fiber: 2.1 g, Total Fat: 33.4 g, Total Carbs: 46.5 g, Protein: 32.3 g

Ingredients

....

2 cups zucchini noodles, spaghetti circles cut

6 cups chicken stock

2 14-oz. cans roasted tomatoes

4 boneless, skinless chicken breasts

5 large garlic cloves, minced

1 yellow onion, chopped

1 large bunch cilantro, chopped (approximately 1 cup)

1 jalapeno pepper, seeded and minced

2 medium carrots, chopped into "coins"

Juice of 2 limes

2 Tbsp. olive oil

1 tsp. cumin

1 tsp. turmeric

1 tsp. black pepper

....

Method

- In a large stock pot, heat the onion, carrots, and garlic in the oil until the onions are translucent.
- Add the canned tomatoes (juice and all), the chicken stock and the chicken pieces. Bring to a boil and cook until the chicken is cooked through. Remove the chicken from the pot and set aside to cool.
- Reduce to a simmer and cover. When the chicken is cool, shred it and return it to the pot, along with the noodles, the spices, and the line juice.
- Continue to simmer for another 30 seconds, then remove from heat.

miso noodle soup (gf/p/wl/v/vg)

This light vegetable/noodle broth can serve as a first course or as a light lunch all by itself.

Prep Time: 25–30 m

Serves: 6–8

Calories: 159, Sodium: 692 mg, Dietary Fiber: 3.9 g, Total Fat: 6.1 g, Total Carbs: 20.2 g, Protein: 7.9 g

Ingredients

....

1 cup zucchini noodles, udon cut

4 carrots, spaghetti cut

3 quarts water

2 leeks, white part only, sliced

1 bunch Swiss chard (or black kale), about ½ pound

4 carrots, cut into chunks

3 cloves garlic, minced

2 green onions, sliced

1 cup edamame (can use frozen)

½ cup miso paste

1 ½ Tbsp. olive oil

....

Method

- Heat the oil in a large stock pot for 1 minute, then add the leeks and garlic. Cook over medium heat for another 5 minutes, stirring occasionally.
- Separate the chard leaves from the ribs and stalks and set aside. Chop the ribs and stalks, then add to the leek and garlic mixture. Continue to cook until the chard is tender, 8-10 minutes. Stir occasionally so the vegetables don't stick.
- Add the water to the pot and bring to a boil. Add the chopped carrots and reduce heat to a simmer. Simmer for 5 minutes or until the carrots are almost soft.
- Chop the chard leaves and add to the soup along with the edamame. Simmer until the greens wilt, then bring to a boil.
- Remove 1 cup of boiling water and add it to the miso paste. Add the miso mixture to the soup along with the noodles and return to a boil. As soon as the noodles are tender (about 30-60 seconds), remove from heat and serve. Garnish with sliced green onions.

Note: You can add chopped chicken or pork to this soup for a heartier version, or diced tofu for a more protein-rich vegetarian/vegan option.

beef pho (gl/p/wl)

Considered the national dish of Vietnam, Pho is traditionally made with beef broth, sometimes enriched with oxtail. This is a simplified version that replaced flat rice noodles with veggie pasta.

Prep Time: 25–30 m

Serves: 4

Calories: 283, Sodium: 2279 mg, Dietary Fiber: 3.2 g, Total Fat: 10.1 g, Total Carbs: 10.8 g, Protein: 35.7 g

Ingredients

....

2 cups yellow squash noodles, udon cut

8 cups beef broth, preferably low sodium

4 cups water

¾ pound flank steak, very thinly sliced

1 medium yellow onion, sliced

4-6 garlic cloves, minced

1 2-inch piece ginger root, grated

2 whole cloves

1 cinnamon stick

2 Tbsp. fish sauce

For garnish: chopped green onions, thinly sliced jalapeno peppers, chopped cilantro, lime wedges

....

Method

- Combine broth, water, and spices in a large stockpot. Bring to a boil over high heat, then cover the pan and reduce the heat. Simmer for half an hour, stirring occasionally.
- Add the noodles and beef to the pot, return to a boil just long enough to cook the beef, about 1-2 minutes if the beef is sliced very thin. Remove the cinnamon stick, then serve hot with garnishes as desired.

minestrone (gf/v/wl)

One of the first Italian words a diner learns (right after "spaghetti," is "minestrone." This classic vegetable soup easily fits into any eating plan that embraces veggies.

Prep Time: 6 h

Serves: 4–6

Calories: 356, Sodium: 810 mg, Dietary Fiber: 24.4 g, Total Fat: 2.0 g, Total Carbs: 61.7 g, Protein: 24.5 g

. . . .

1 cup zucchini or yellow squash pasta, spaghetti circles cut

4 cups chicken broth

1 28-oz. can crushed tomatoes

1 15.5-oz. can cannellini beans, drained and rinsed to remove excess salt

1 cup escarole or kale, shredded

2 large carrots, cut into "coins"

2 ribs celery, diced

1 large yellow onion, chopped

3 large garlic cloves, minced

2 tsp. Italian seasoning

Grated Parmesan cheese (optional)

. . . .

Method

- Combine the broth and the canned tomatoes (juice included) with the carrots, celery, garlic, and onion in a slow cooker. Stir in the Italian seasoning. (If using tomatoes that have "Italian seasoning" don't add more.)
- Cover and cook on low for 4-6 hours, then add the escarole, and beans. Cover and increase heat. Cook for another 5-10 minutes, until the greens are wilted.
- Add the noodles and cook another 1-2 minutes. Serve hot, garnished with Parmesan if desired.

Note: Without the Parmesan garnish, this recipe is Paleo; substitute vegetable broth for the chicken broth to make it vegan.

pasta e fagilo (gf/p)

This pasta and bean soup is another hearty, healthy example of "Mediterranean" cuisine. Substitute short, curly zucchini noodles made with the Paderno for the traditional tiny tube-shaped pasta.

Prep Time: 45 m

Serves: 8

Calories: 549, Sodium: 1046 mg, Dietary Fiber: 24.2 g, Total Fat: 11.0 g, Total Carbs: 76.5 g, Protein: 38.9 g

Ingredients

....

1 cup zucchini or yellow squash pasta, flat semicircles cut

1 pound spicy Italian sausage (if using links, remove casing)

4 cups chicken broth

1 cup water

4 carrots, sliced into coins

1 large yellow onion, diced

4 cloves garlic, crushed

1 16-oz. can tomato sauce

1 15-oz. can diced tomatoes

1 15-oz. can kidney beans

1 15-oz can cannellini or navy beans

1 Tbsp. Italian seasoning

....

Method

- Crumble the sausage into the bottom of a large stockpot or Dutch oven and brown over medium heat. Drain off the excess fat and then add the olive oil, garlic, onions, and carrots. Cook until the vegetables are tender (about 4 minutes). Stir occasionally.
- Add the water, chicken stock, tomato sauce, and diced tomatoes (including juice). Stir in the Italian seasoning and bring to a boil.
- Drain and rinse the canned beans, then add to the soup. Add the beans to the pot and reduce heat. Simmer for 2-3 minutes, then toss in the noodles and simmer another 1-2 minutes. Serve hot.

sizzling "rice" soup (gf/p)

Substituting cauliflower for the rice in this recipe gives it an extra layer of flavor as well as converting it into a dish that's gluten-free and paleo.

Prep Time: 25–30 m

Serves: 8

Calories: 579, Sodium: 374 mg, Dietary Fiber: __, Total Fat: 56.5 g, Total Carbs: 6.0 g, Protein: 11.8 g

Ingredients

....

2/3 cup cauliflower, "rice" cut

3 cups chicken broth

¼ cup baby shrimp (can use canned or frozen)

1 boneless, skinless chicken breast cut into bite-sized pieces

2 Tbsp. chopped water chestnuts

¼ cup bamboo shoots

½ cup mushrooms, sliced

½ cup bean sprouts

1 large egg

2 cups canola oil

1 Tbsp. dry sherry

4 Tbsp. cornstarch

....

Method
- Combine the egg and cornstarch. Add the shrimp and chicken pieces and stir to coat.
- Heat 1 ½ cups oil in a wok.
- Add the chicken and shrimp and quickly stir-fry until cooked through. Remove from oil and set aside.
- In a large saucepan, combine the broth, mushrooms, and bamboo shoots. Bring to a boil.
- Add the sherry, reduce heat and simmer.
- Re-heat the soil in the wok and quickly brown the cauliflower "rice." Remove from the oil and drain. Add the "rice" and bean sprouts to the soup and serve immediately.

pumpkin noodle soup (gf/wl/v/vg)

This soup combines rich fall flavors with an ease of preparation that will make it a favorite.

Prep Time: 25 m

Serves: 6

Calories: 150, Sodium: 645 mg, Dietary Fiber: 6.3 g, Total Fat: 6.3 g, Total Carbs: 19.3 g, Protein: 6.2 g

Ingredients

....

4 cups pumpkin or squash noodles, flat cut

5 cups vegetable broth

1 large (29-oz.) can pumpkin puree (not the pumpkin pie filling kind)

1 large yellow onion, diced

2 Tbsp. olive oil

½ Tbsp. brown sugar

2 tsp. sage (or 2 Tbsp. fresh sage, chopped)

1 tsp. cinnamon

¼ tsp. ginger

¼ tsp. cayenne pepper

1/8 tsp. nutmeg

....

Method

- Heat the oil in a large saucepot and add the chopped onions. Cook until the onions are translucent, 3-5 minutes. Stir in the spices.
- Add the pumpkin puree and the vegetable broth. Bring to a boil, then reduce to a simmer.
- Stir in the brown sugar.
- Add the pumpkin noodles and summer for another 2-3 minutes.
- Note: Leave out the brown sugar to make this soup Paleo-friendly.

moroccan chicken with olives (gf/p)

If you can't find preserved lemons in your local market (try the olive bar), you can substitute fresh lemon peel.

Prep Time: 45 m

Serves: 4

Calories: 1288, Sodium: 3086 mg, Dietary Fiber: 6.3 g, Total Fat: 96.1 g, Total Carbs: 36.3 g, Protein: 68.8 g

Ingredients

....

4 cups zucchini noodles, cooked al dente

2 cups yellow squash noodles, cooked al dente

3 lbs. chicken legs and thighs

3 cups chicken stock

2 preserved lemons (or rind from two fresh lemons)

¾ cup pitted green olives, rinsed

1 small yellow onion, diced

4 Tbsp. coconut oil

1 garlic clove, minced

1 tsp. grated fresh ginger

1 Tbsp. cumin

1 Tbsp. ground coriander

1 tsp, turmeric

2 tsp. paprika

½ tsp. cayenne pepper

¼ tsp. saffron

....

Method

- Remove pulp from the preserved lemons and cut peel into narrow strips. If using fresh lemons, cut the rind into narrow strips. Set the lemon strips aside.
- Combine the squash and zucchini noodles in a medium bowl.
- Melt the coconut oil in a Dutch oven over medium heat. Add the chicken pieces. Season with salt and pepper to taste, then brown on all sides. (Do this in batches if necessary.) Set the browned chicken aside.

- Add the onions to the fat and cook until translucent and slightly softened. Add all the spices except the saffron and stir.
- Return the chicken pieces to the pan and turn until they're coated with the oil/spice mixture.
- Add the chicken stock and the saffron. Stir.
- Cover and Reduce heat. Simmer for 25 minutes.
- Add the lemon strips and olives. Cook for another 5-8 minutes, covered, until the chicken is done.
- Remove the chicken and set aside.
- Bring the sauce to a boil and cook until it thickens slightly, about 10 minutes.
- 1Divide the vegetable noodles among four plates. Top with the hot sauce, then add the chicken.

shrimp soup with bok choy (gf/p/wl)

This seafood soup is half a world away from the tomato-based seafood stews found in the Mediterranean.

Prep Time: 35–45 m

Serves: 6–8

Calories: 307, Sodium: 1066 mg, Dietary Fiber: 1.9 g, Total Fat: 8.3 g, Total Carbs: 27.5 g, Protein: 30.4 g

Ingredients

....

3 cups zucchini pasta, spaghetti cut

1 ½ cups clam juice (or seafood stock)

6 cups chicken stock

2 lbs. raw shrimp, cleaned, shelled, and deveined

1 large bok choy, trimmed and sliced thinly

3 green onions, thinly sliced

1 Tbsp. crushed red pepper flakes

2 Tbsp. grated ginger

3 large garlic cloves, minced

1/3 lb. shiitake mushrooms, sliced

3 Tbsp. canola oil

....

Method

- Heat the oil in a large stockpot and add the bok choy, mushrooms, garlic, ginger, and red pepper flakes. Heat on medium for a minute, then add the broth and clam juice. Cover the pot and bring to a boil.
- Add the shrimp and sliced green onions. Continue to cook for another 2 minutes, or until shrimp are cooked through.
- Toss in the noodles, remove from heat and let stand 5 minutes before serving.

black bean & noodle soup (gf/wl/v/vg)

This festive and flavorful soup is high-fiber and low-calorie, and makes an excellent starter for a Cinco de Mayo feast or a treat to kick off an ordinary weekend.

Prep Time: 25 m

Serves: 6

Calories: 334, Sodium: 887 mg, Dietary Fiber: 13.8 g, Total Fat: 2.4 g, Total Carbs: 61.5 g, Protein: 21.0 g

Ingredients

....

2 cups zucchini or yellow squash noodles, spaghetti cut

2 14-oz. cans vegetable broth

1 16-oz. jar salsa

1 15-oz can black beans, drained and rinsed

2 cups corn kernels (preferably frozen, not canned)

Juice of one lime

1-2 tsp. chili powder

½ tsp. cumin

....

Method

- Heat the broth to a boil in a medium saucepan.
- Add the remaining ingredients.

- Continue to cook for 1-2 minutes, until noodles are tender.

Note: Feel free to garnish with a dollop of sour cream if not following a vegan diet.

CHAPTER 5

SALADS

At formal dinners salads are served as a separate course while at family-style meals they're usually served on the side. Hearty or light, warm or cold, these salads will add the finishing touch to your menu.

greek pasta salad (gf/wl)

The Greek flavors of this quick and easy pasta salad make a nice change from the more common "Italian" versions.

Prep Time: 15 m

Serves: 4–6

Calories: 410, Sodium: 537 mg, Dietary Fiber: 3.1 g, Total Fat: 27.0 g, Total Carbs: 33 g, Protein: 11.1 g

Ingredients

....

4 cups zucchini pasta, udon circles cut

1 bunch green onions, sliced

1 basket cherry tomatoes, halved

1 pkg. sliced white mushrooms

1 large bell pepper, seeded and sliced into matchsticks

1 4-oz. can pitted black olives, drained

¾ cup pepperoni, thinly sliced

1 cup feta cheese, crumbled

2 large garlic cloves, minced

2 tsp. basil

1 ½ tsp. oregano

½ tsp. black pepper

½ cup olive oil

½ cup red wine vinegar

....

Method
- Blanche the noodles if you desire a softer noodle. Otherwise leave raw.
- In a large bowl, combine the oil, vinegar, garlic, basil, oregano, and pepper. Whisk to blend.
- Add remaining ingredients, including noodles, and toss to distribute dressing evenly.
- Chill overnight to blend flavors.

Note: Leave out the pepperoni to convert this to a vegetarian salad.

asian chicken & noodle salad (gf/wl)

Chicken and noodles served in a salad rather than a soup. Since peanuts and peanut butter are off the menu for GF diets, consider making this with almond butter for a change.

Prep Time: 1 h 20 m

Serves: 4

Calories: 551, Sodium: 1,523 mg, Dietary Fiber: 6.2 g, Total Fat: 19.9 g, Total Carbs: 55 g, Protein: 39.8 g

Ingredients

....

3 cups zucchini or yellow squash noodles, flat cut

2 cups cooked chicken breast cut in bite-size pieces

½ cup creamy peanut butter

3 Tbsp. water

4 Tbsp. gluten-free soy sauce

3 Tbsp. rice vinegar

2 Tbsp. chili-garlic sauce

2 Tbsp. grated fresh ginger

1 Tbsp. light brown sugar

1 small bunch cilantro, leaves only chopped

1 bunch green onions, sliced thin

2 medium carrots grated

1 bell pepper, cut in matchsticks

....

Method

- Blanche the noodles if you desire a softer noodle. Otherwise leave raw.
- In a large serving bowl, combine the noodles, chicken, grated carrots, bell pepper, cilantro, and green onions.
- In a food processor or blender, combine the peanut butter, soy sauce, chili-garlic sauce, brown sugar, and water. Blend until smooth. If the dressing is too thick, add a little more water.
- Pour dressing over salad and toss to coat. Chill for an hour.

mediterranean pasta salad (gf/p)

This is more of a pasta side dish than a salad. If you want the ingredients to "stick together" more, you can replace 2 Tbsp. of the olive oil with mayonnaise or Greek yogurt—it just won't be Paleo any more.

Prep Time: 12 m

Serves: 4

Calories: 176, Sodium: 55 mg, Dietary Fiber: 1.0 g, Total Fat: 5.8 g, Total Carbs: 17.8 g, Protein: 14.0 g

Ingredients

....

4 cups zucchini, spaghetti cut

2 cups cooked chicken breast, cut in bite-sized pieces

3 hard-boiled egg whites, diced

1 small red onion, diced

2 garlic cloves, minced

3 Tbsp. olive oil

Juice of ½ lemon

1 tsp. basil

½ tsp. dried rosemary

Sliced black olives (for garnish)

....

Method

- Blanche the noodles if you desire a softer noodle. Otherwise leave raw.
- Combine the noodles, chicken, diced egg whites, and red onion in a small bowl.
- Combine the other ingredients and whisk to blend well. Pour over the noodle/chicken mixture and toss to blend.
- Garnish with sliced olives if desired.

Note: Can also garnish with some crumbled feta cheese if not Paleo.

spicy slaw (gf/wl/v/vg)

This mayonnaise-free slaw is light and lively with a dash of hot pepper sauce to give it some bite. Try it without the sugar to make the recipe Paleo-friendly.

Prep Time: 75 m

Serves: 4–6

Calories: 95, Sodium: 30 mg, Dietary Fiber: 2.0 g, Total Fat: 7.1 g, Total Carbs: 7.9 g, Protein: 0.9 g

Ingredients

....

4 cups green cabbage, shredded

3 carrots, spaghetti cut

3 Tbsp. apple cider vinegar

3 Tbsp. olive oil

1 Tbsp. granulated sugar

½ tsp. dry mustard

¼ tsp. pepper

½ tsp. hot pepper sauce (or to taste)

....

Method

- Combine the shredded cabbage and carrot noodles.
- Combine all the other ingredients with a whisk. Pour over the cabbage and carrots.
- Refrigerate for at least an hour to blend flavors.

mexican slaw (gf/p/wl/v/vg)

This variation on a theme salad pairs cabbage with radishes and poblano chilies. If you like more heat, use substitute a hotter pepper like a jalapeno or serrano.

Prep Time: 10 m

Serves: 4–6

Calories: 75, Sodium: 35 mg, Dietary Fiber: 1.6 g, Total Fat: 3.4 g, Total Carbs: 10.3 g, Protein: 1.1 g

Ingredients

....

1/2 small head green cabbage, shredded

1/2 small head Napa cabbage, shredded

1 small bunch red radishes

2 fresh poblano chilies (or Hatch chiles)

Juice of three limes

1 Tbsp. canola oil

1 bunch fresh cilantro, minced (about 2 cups)

¼ tp. Cayenne pepper

....

Method

- Remove tough outer leaves from cabbage and cut out core. (This won't be necessary if using a Paderno slicer.) Shred the cabbage.
- Trim the radishes and slice thinly.
- De-seed the peppers and cut into small dice.
- Mix the cabbages, radishes, and peppers in a large bowl and set aside.
- Mix together the lime juice and pepper. Add the cilantro and let sit for 5 minutes. Whisk in the soil. Pour vinaigrette over the vegetables and toss to blend. Either serve immediately, or chill for an hour.

jerusalem artichoke slaw (gf/v)

Cooked Jerusalem artichokes can sub for potatoes in a lot of dishes; served raw as they are here, they have a crisp texture reminiscent of water chestnuts.

Prep Time: 75 m

Serves: 4–6

Calories: 94, Sodium: 34 mg, Dietary Fiber: 1.0 g, Total Fat: 2.3 g, Total Carbs: 10.9 g, Protein: 7.8 g

Ingredients

....

1 large carrot, matchstick cut

½ lb. Jerusalem artichokes, peeled, matchstick cut

2 Tbsp. sour cream

2 Tbsp. Greek yogurt

1 Tsp. dry mustard

2 tsp. white wine vinegar

¼ tsp. black pepper

....

Method
- Chopped parsley (if desired) for garnish
- Combine the sour cream, yogurt, mustard, and vinegar. Add pepper.
- Pour dressing over the vegetables. Chill for an hour to blend flavors.

colorful carrot & beet slaw (gf/p/v/vg)

This colorful slaw substitutes beets and carrots for the more common cabbage and uses a basic vinaigrette as the dressing instead of mayonnaise.

Prep Time: 15 m

Serves: 4

Calories: 161, Sodium: 197 mg, Dietary Fiber: 3.7 g, Total Fat: 11.0 g, Total Carbs: 15.4 g, Protein: 2.2 g

....

3 large beets, spaghetti cut

4 large carrots, spaghetti cut

2 Tbsp. Dijon mustard

3 Tbsp. red wine vinegar

3 Tbsp. olive oil

1 tsp. black pepper

....

Method

- Place beet and carrot noodles into a plate.
- Combine oil, vinegar, mustard, and pepper. Pour vinaigrette over noodles. Garnish with parsley.

dilled salmon pasta salad (gf/v)

This is a good recipe to make a little salmon go a long way and a tasty alternative to the traditional tuna salad option.

Prep Time: 20 m

Serves: 6

Calories: 676, Sodium: 192 mg, Dietary Fiber: 4.0 g, Total Fat: 40.0 g, Total Carbs: 58.4 g, Protein: 24.5 g

Ingredients

....

8 cups zucchini pasta, spaghetti circles cut

1 15-oz can salmon, drained and flaked

1 bunch fresh dill, minced

2 bell peppers, seeded and minced (can use any color)

1 cup olive oil

1/3 cup Dijon mustard

½ red wine vinegar

2 cloves garlic, minced

....

Method
- Blanche the zucchini noodles if a soft noodle is desired, otherwise leave uncooked.
- Whisk the olive oil with the mustard, garlic, and vinegar in a large bowl.
- Add the noodles, peppers, and salmon.
- Toss to combine.

noodles & humus salad (gf)

This cross-cultural dish—originally made with Soba noodles—is a fresh take on pasta salad that's perfect for a light lunch or as a dinner side.

Prep Time: 10 m

Serves: 4

Calories: 454, Sodium: 1107 mg, Dietary Fiber: 5.7 g, Total Fat: 213 g, Total Carbs: 54.6 g, Protein: 11.4 g

Ingredients

....

4 cups zucchini noodles, udon cut

2 medium carrots, udon cut

¾ cup prepared humus (classic, not flavored)

1 bell pepper, seeded and diced

3 green onions, thinly sliced

¼ cup canola oil

1 tsp. dark sesame oil

4 Tbsp. soy sauce

4 Tbsp. rice vinegar

1 tsp. ginger

2 Tbsp. fresh mint

1 tsp. crushed red pepper flakes

....

Method

- Blanche the carrot noodles. If you like soft zucchini noodles, then blanche the zucchini, otherwise leave uncooked.
- Combine the noodles with the peppers, and green onions in a large bowl.
- Combine the oil, vinegar, herbs, and spices. Mix well and pour over the noodle/vegetable combination.
- Stir in the humus and toss to blend.

thai green papaya salad (gf/wl/v/vg)

This traditional Thai salad is a refreshing blend of sweet and hot, with a salty accent of fish sauce.

Prep Time: 20–25 m

Serves: 4

Calories: 451, Sodium: 785 mg, Dietary Fiber: 6.2 g, Total Fat: 17.1 g, Total Carbs: 69.5 g, Protein: 12.2 g

Ingredients

....

2 green papayas, peeled, spaghetti cut

2 medium carrots, spaghetti cut

2 cups bean sprouts

10 grape tomatoes, cut in half

½ cup fresh basil, chopped roughly

½ cup unsalted peanuts, chopped coarsely

2 Tbsp. canola oil

½ tsp. soy sauce

2 Tbsp. fish sauce

Juice of two limes

....

Method

- Mix the papaya, carrots, tomatoes, and chopped basil.
- Combine the oil, soy sauce, fish sauce, and lime juice. Pour the dressing over the salad and toss to combine.
- Garnish with chopped peanuts.

Note: substitute almonds for the peanuts to convert this to a Paleo recipe.

CHAPTER 6

SIDES

Think about your most memorable meals—often it wasn't the entrees that had you salivating, it was the dishes on the side. Why not make some memories with these recipes?

vegetables with rosemary vinaigrette (gf/p/wl/v/vg)

This is a great winter side dish that's easy to make with a vegetable spiralizer or julienne slicer.

Prep Time: 40 m

Serves: 8–10

Calories: 229, Sodium: 53 mg, Dietary Fiber: 7.8 g, Total Fat: 5.1 g, Total Carbs: 43.8 g, Protein: 3.6 g

Ingredients

....

4 carrots, julienne sliced

2 turnips, julienne sliced

4 yellow squash, julienne sliced

2 medium sweet potatoes, julienne sliced

2 bell peppers, de-seeded and julienne sliced

1 large yellow onion, thinly sliced

1 bunch fresh rosemary, coarsely chopped

4 leaves fresh sage, chopped (or 1 tsp. dried sage)

1 Tablespoon Italian seasoning

3 large garlic cloves, minced

3 Tbsp. balsamic vinegar

1 tsp. black pepper

3 Tbsp. olive oil

....

Method

- Heat the olive oil in a large skillet and sauté the vegetables until they are crisp/tender.
- Combine the vinegar and remaining ingredients and pour over the vegetables in the skillet.
- Cook for another 5 minutes to blend flavors.

Note: A variation on this dish is roasted vegetables with rosemary vinaigrette. Place all the vegetables in a large baking pan. Combine the oil and vinegar and spices as if for salad dressing. Pour over the vegetables and bake for an hour at 400 degrees or until the vegetables are tender.

squash sauté (gf/wl/v)

Mix and match yellow squash and zucchini for a more colorful dish.

Prep Time: 25–30 m

Serves: 8

Calories: 100, Sodium: 39 mg, Dietary Fiber: 2.2 g, Total Fat: 6.9 g, Total Carbs: 8.5 g, Protein: 2.9 g

Ingredients

....

2 lbs. summer squash, matchstick or spaghetti circles cut

1 lb. ripe Roma tomatoes, thinly sliced

1 medium yellow onion, thinly sliced

3 Tbsp. olive oil

2 large garlic cloves, minced

½ tsp. crushed dried red pepper flakes

1 Tbsp. Italian seasoning

Parmesan cheese for garnish

....

Method

- Heat the oil in a large skillet. Sauté the onion and garlic until the onion is translucent.
- Add the tomatoes and sauté until the tomatoes have released their juices.
- Add the squash and sauté for another 1-2 minutes.
- Stir in the Italian seasoning and the pepper flakes.
- Serve hot.
- Garnish with parmesan cheese if desired.

bleu cheese & spinach pasta (gf/v)

This is another chameleon of a dish that can do double-duty as a side or a salad, depending on the number of diners.

Prep Time: 25 m

Serves: 6

Calories: 153, Sodium: 411 mg, Dietary Fiber: 1.1 g, Total Fat: 12.7 g, Total Carbs: 4.1 g, Protein: 6.1 g

Ingredients

....

3 cups zucchini or yellow squash pasta, spaghetti circles cut

4 oz. bleu cheese, crumbled

1 large bunch spinach, chopped coarsely

1 small red onion, sliced into rings

1 cup vegetable broth

2 Tbsp. balsamic vinegar (may substitute red wine vinegar)

3 Tbsp. olive oil

½ tsp. black pepper

....

Method

- Using a large skillet, heat the onions in 1 Tbsp. oil until they are beginning to brown.
- Combine the broth, the vinegar, the black pepper and the chopped spinach and add to the pan. Cook for 3 minutes until the spinach has wilted.
- Add the noodles and the cheese, stir to combine and cook until the cheese is melted, about 5 minutes.

florentine potato pasta casserole (gf)

This cheesy potato casserole is a great "transition" dish, offering the comforting combo of potatoes and cheese with the nutritional punch of spinach. Add some chopped leftover chicken or ham to make it a main meal.

Prep Time: 90 m

Serves: 6

Calories: 247, Sodium: 689 mg, Dietary Fiber: 3.3 g, Total Fat: 8.8 g, Total Carbs: 30.6 g, Protein: 14.2 g

Ingredients

....

4 cups baking potatoes, julienned or flat cut

1 package sliced mushrooms (about 2 cups)

4 cups chicken broth

1 medium yellow onion, chopped

1 large garlic clove, minced

1 10-oz package frozen chopped spinach, thawed and drained and squeezed dry

2 ½ cups milk (can use low fat)

1 Tbsp. olive oil

1/3 cup shredded cheese of choice

½ tsp. black pepper

Parmesan cheese for garnish.

Method

- Preheat oven to 350 degrees.
- Coat a baking dish (approx 11 x 7) with butter, oil, or non-stick cooking spray.
- In a large skillet, heat the onions, mushrooms, and garlic in the olive oil until the onion is translucent and the onions have started to "shrivel."
- Add the broth and black pepper. Continue to sauté over medium-high heat until the broth has been absorbed or evaporated.
- Stir in the spinach.
- Begin layering the potatoes into the prepared baking dish. Cover with a layer of the spinach/mushroom mixture.
- Cover with 1/2 of the cheese mixture.
- Add another layer of potatoes and the rest of the spinach mixture.
- Combine the milk and eggs and cornstarch.
- Pour over the layers, making sure everything is moist.
- Bake in the pre-heated over for 1 hour.
- Top the casserole with the rest of the cheese and bake for another 15-20 minutes until the cheese is bubbling and golden brown.
- Garnish with parmesan cheese if desired.
- Remove from oven and let sit for 5 minutes before serving.

Note: Use "pepperjack"' Monterey Jack cheese to give this casserole a little kick.

sesame noodles (gf/v/vg)

This recipe is the "little black dress" of cuisine. As is, it's a hearty side dish or light lunch. Add a little sautéed tofu and a package of frozen "Asian" vegetables for a vegetarian entrée.

Prep Time: 20 m

Serves: 8

Calories: 253, Sodium: 25 mg, Dietary Fiber: 1.4 g, Total Fat: 13.7 g, Total Carbs: 28.3 g, Protein: 4.5 g

Ingredients

....

4 cups zucchini or yellow squash noodles, udon cut

1 bunch green onions, sliced thin

4 large garlic cloves, minced

3 Tbsp. honey

¼ cup gluten-free soy sauce

1/3 cup rice vinegar

1/3 cup canola oil

2 Tbsp. dark sesame oil

1 Tbsp. crushed red pepper

1 Tbsp. toasted sesame seeds

....

Method
- Place the noodles in a large serving bowl.
- Combine the canola and sesame oil, vinegar, soy sauce, and honey in a small saucepan and bring to a boil. Add the crushed red pepper.
- Pour hot mixture over the noodles. Toss to coat.
- Garnish with sliced green onions and sesame seeds.

veggie pasta with bacon and swiss chard (gf)

This rustic combination of pasta, bacon and greens is a mainstay of Mediterranean cooking.

Prep Time: 25–30 m

Serves: 4

Calories: 616, Sodium: 2,116 mg, Dietary Fiber: 2.5 g, Total Fat: 47.7 g, Total Carbs: 10.3 g, Protein: 35.9 g

Ingredients

....

4 cups zucchini or yellow squash pasta, spaghetti cut

¾ pound bacon, cut into ½-inch slices

1 large yellow onion, sliced thinly

2 large bunches Swiss chard, stemmed, ribs removed, and chopped

3 Tbsp. olive oil

2 Tbsp. balsamic vinegar

¾ cup grated Parmesan cheese

....

Method

- Blanche the noodles, and reserve 1 cup of pasta-cooking liquid. Place the cooked pasta in a large serving bowl.
- Fry the bacon in a large, heavy skillet until it is beginning to crisp (about 10 minutes). Remove bacon from pan and drain on paper towels.
- Remove all but 3 tablespoons of bacon fat from skillet.
- Add onion and sauté over medium heat until soft and translucent. Add the chard and the reserved pasta-cooking liquid.
- Stir to combine and cook until the chard is wilted.
- Pour over the pasta.
- Crumble the bacon and sprinkle over the pasta.
- Garnish with the cheese.

Note: Eliminate the Parmesan cheese to make this dish Paleo-friendly as well as vegan.

noodle kugel (gf/v)

Is it a side dish or a dessert? Depends on the occasion and the amount of sugar added.

Prep Time: 80 m

Serves: 8–10

Calories: 199, Sodium: 166 mg, Dietary Fiber: __, Total Fat: 11.6 g, Total Carbs: 16.9 g, Protein: 7.8 g

Ingredients

....

2 cups zucchini noodles, udon cut

1 8-oz. container cottage cheese

1 8-oz. container sour cream

1 ½ cups milk

½ stick butter, melted

2 eggs

¼ cup granulated sugar

....

Method

- Preheat oven to 350 degrees.
- In a large mixing bowl, combine the cottage cheese, sour cream, butter, eggs, sugar, and milk.
- Add the noodles and mix well.
- Coat a glass baking pan (approx 13 x 9) with butter or non-stick spray and fill with the noodle mixture.
- Bake for an hour at 375 until browned on top.

Note: To make a sweeter dessert kugel, increase the sugar to 2/3 cup and add 1 tsp. vanilla extract.

CHAPTER 7

ENTREES

The entrée is the main course, the base a meal is built upon. If you take away all the extras, what you're left with is the entrée.

pasta with lemon & ricotta (gf/wl/v)

In Italy, pasta is often served in small portions as a separate course; feel free to repurpose this creamy pasta dish as a side.

Prep Time: 20 m

Serves: 2

Calories: 672, Sodium: 263 mg, Dietary Fiber: 5.1 g, Total Fat: 22.6 g, Total Carbs: 91.6 g, Protein: 30.1 g

Ingredients

....

4 cups zucchini or yellow squash pasta, spaghetti cut

2 quarts water

1 8-oz. container ricotta cheese

¼ stick butter, cut into pieces

½ cup chopped flat-leaf parsley

½ tsp. black pepper

Zest from one lemon

....

Method

- Bring the water to boil in a large saucepan.
- Boil the pasta for 1-2 minutes until tender. Remove 1 cup of water from the pasta pot.
- Combine the cheese, butter and reserved pasta water, whisking until creamy.
- Drain the pasta and put in a large serving bowl.
- Add the parsley, pepper, lemon zest and the cream toss.
- Toss with tongs to mix.

Serve immediately.

greek lamb pasta (gf/p/wl)

Lamb is an increasingly economical option as chicken prices soar and it pairs well with pasta.

Prep Time: 50–60 m

Serves: 4–6

Calories: 380, Sodium: 267 mg, Dietary Fiber: 6.6 g, Total Fat: 9.2 g, Total Carbs: 45.4 g, Protein: 30.2 g

Ingredients

....

4 cups zucchini or yellow squash noodles, flat cut

1 lb. ground lamb

1 4-oz can sliced black olives, drained

1 28-oz. can diced tomatoes

1 small can tomato paste (leave out for Paleo diets)

2 Tbsp. oregano (or Greek seasoning blend)

3 large garlic cloves, minced

1 large yellow onion, diced

1 large bell pepper, diced

Juice of one lemon

3 Tbsp. balsamic vinegar

....

Method

- In a large saucepan brown the ground lamb. Add the onion, bell pepper, garlic and olives and cook until the onions become translucent.
- Add the diced tomatoes, lemon juice, vinegar, and spices.
- Simmer for 10 minutes, then stir in tomato paste.
- Simmer another 10-20 minutes, adding small amounts of water if the sauce becomes too thick.
- Ladle over the pasta, wait several minutes to allow the pasta to soften, then serve.

Note: If not following a Paleo diet, sprinkle with a little feta cheese before serving.

eggplant pasta sauce (gf/p/wl)

This sauce is spectacular when made with young, tender "baby" eggplants and is a good dish to introduce the vegetable to skeptics. Put it together in the morning and it'll be ready when you come home from work.

Prep Time: 8 h 15 m

Serves: 2

Calories: 835, Sodium: 840 mg, Dietary Fiber: 47.7 g, Total Fat: 5.2 g, Total Carbs: 171.1 g, Protein: 32.4 g

Ingredients

………………………………………

4 cups zucchini pasta, flat circles cut

4 small ("baby") eggplants or one large one

1 medium yellow onion, chopped

1 28-oz. can Italian-style plum tomatoes

3 large garlic cloves, chopped

1 4-oz can sliced mushrooms, drained

1/3 cup dry red wine

1/3 cup water

1 ½ tsp. Italian seasoning

………………………………………

Method

- Peel eggplant and dice into 1-inch cubes.
- Combine all the ingredients except the pasta and olives in a 5 ½ quart slow cooker.
- Cook on low-heat setting for 8 hours.
- Boil 2 quarts of water in a large saucepan. Blanche the pasta and drain.
- Stir the olives into the sauce.
- Divide the hot pasta onto plates and top with sauce.

turkey pie with spaghetti crust (gf/v)

The veggie spaghetti crust can be adapted to work with any quiche. It is cheese-heavy, though, so it's not suitable for Paleo or Weight-loss diets.

Prep Time: 55 m

Serves: 4

Calories: 408, Sodium: 561 mg, Dietary Fiber: 2.4 g, Total Fat: 18.9 g, Total Carbs: 29.8 g, Protein: 32.3 g

Ingredients

....

2 cups zucchini noodles, spaghetti cut

¼ pound ground turkey

¼ stick butter

1 egg, beaten

¼ cup fresh grated Parmesan cheese

1 cup cottage cheese

2 tbsp. butter, divided

1 egg, beaten

2 tbsp. grated Parmesan cheese

2/3 c. low fat cottage cheese

1/2 c. each diced onion & green pepper

5 oz. cooked ground turkey, crumbled

1 c. canned Italian tomatoes (with liquid), drained & chopped, reserving liquid

1/4 c. tomato sauce

1 tsp. each sugar & oregano

1/2 tsp. salt

Dash each garlic powder & pepper

4 oz. Mozzarella cheese, shredded

....

Method

- Preheat oven to 350 degrees.
- Coat 9" pie pan with butter or non-stick cooking spray and set aside. Melt 1 tablespoon butter.
- In 1 quart bowl combine spaghetti, egg, Parmesan cheese and melted butter, mixing well.
- Press spaghetti mixture over bottom and up sides of sprayed pan to form a crust. Spread cottage cheese over crust.
- In skillet heat remaining butter; add onion and green pepper and sauté until soft.
- Add remaining ingredients except Mozzarella cheese and stir to combine.
- Reduce heat and simmer about ten minutes.
- Spread mixture evenly over cottage cheese and bake 15 to 20 minutes. Sprinkle pie with Mozzarella and bake until lightly brown, about 5 minutes longer.
- Remove from oven and let stand 5 minutes before slicing.

smoked salmon pasta with lemon & dill (gf/v)

This delicious pasta works as the centerpiece for a Sunday brunch or as a light supper with a side salad and a nice glass of the white wine used in the sauce.

Prep Time: 25 m

Serves: 2

Calories: 902, Sodium: 1282 mg, Dietary Fiber: 12.6 g, Total Fat: 32.1 g, Total Carbs: 111.1 g, Protein: 36.0 g

Ingredients

....

4 cups zucchini or yellow squash noodles, udon cut

1 4-oz. package smoked salmon, cut in strips

½ cup dry white wine

¼ cup fresh dill, chopped

1 small red onion, minced

3 Tbsp. olive oil

½ cup and half

1 8-oz package frozen peas, thawed and drained

1 lemon, cut in wedges

....

Method

- Blanche noodles, drain and place in a large bowl.
- In a large skillet, heat the oil and sauté the onion until it is soft and translucent.
- Add the white wine to the skillet, reduce heat, and simmer until it is reduced in volume and beginning to thicken.
- Add the peas and then the half and half, stirring gently.
- Simmer for 3 more minutes, then add the salmon and dill.
- Heat through and stir until the sauce has thickened a little more.
- Pour the sauce over the pasta in the serving bowl and toss to blend.
- Serve immediately, garnished with lemon wedges.

Note: This dish can be made with canned or leftover poached salmon if you prefer.

pasta with anchovy sauce (gf/p)

The anchovies in this sauce dissolve in the oil and leave just their salty, fishy essence behind.

Prep Time: 10–15 m

Serves: 4–6

Calories: 365, Sodium: 1,409 mg, Dietary Fiber: 1.2 g, Total Fat: 36.9 g, Total Carbs: 3.9 g, Protein: 7.1 g

....

4 cups zucchini or yellow squash noodles, spaghetti cut

12 anchovy filets, packed in olive oil (2-ounce can)

1 cup olive oil

1 Tbsp. crushed red pepper flakes

Juice from one lemon

¼ cup Italian parsley, minced

....

Method

- Drain oil and mince anchovies.
- In a small saucepan, heat the minced anchovies in ½ cup olive oil. Stir until the fish "melt" into the oil (about 5 minutes).
- Stir in the pepper flakes and the rest of the olive oil.
- Add the lemon juice and stir.
- Pour the hot sauce over the raw noodles and mix together.

beef ragu over potato pasta (gf/p/wl)

Try this new combination of meat and potatoes as a change of pace. Substitute zucchini pasta for the potatoes to make the recipe low carb.

Prep Time: 55 m

Serves: 4

Calories: 520, Sodium: 84 mg, Dietary Fiber: 7.7 g, Total Fat: 20.6 g, Total Carbs: 55.6 g, Protein: 23.7 g

Ingredients

....

4 cups zucchini or yellow squash noodles, flat cut

1 ½ pounds ground beef or turkey

1 large yellow onion, chopped coarsely

3 large garlic cloves, minced

1/3 cup dry red wine

2 14 ½ ounce cans "Italian style" diced tomato

1 large carrot, coarsely chopped

2 Tbsp. Italian seasoning

1/3 cup half and half

2 Tbsp. olive oil

Grated Parmesan cheese for garnish

....

Method

- Heat oil in a large saucepan. Add the meat, onion, garlic, and carrot. Sauté until meat is no longer pink, about 8 minutes. Add wine and cook for 3-5 minutes until it evaporates, stirring constantly. Stir in the tomatoes (juice included) the half and half and the Italian seasoning.
- Reduce heat, cover the pan and simmer until the sauce has thickened (about 25 minutes).
- When the sauce is done, ladle it over the zucchini noodles to "cook" them.
- Garnish with parmesan cheese if desired (and not following Paleo).

pasta puttanesca (gf/p/wl)

This is another classic Italian pasta sauce that is fast and easy to make, yet still full of big flavors.

Prep Time: 30 m

Serves: 2–4

Calories: 413, Sodium: 537 mg, Dietary Fiber: 9.6 g, Total Fat: 8.9 g, Total Carbs: 61.9 g, Protein: 23.5 g

Ingredients

....

4 cups zucchini or yellow squash pasta, spaghetti cut

6 anchovies canned in oil (half a 2-oz. can)

1 28-oz. can crushed tomatoes

½ cup pitted black olives, chopped

2 Tbsp. tomato paste

4 garlic cloves, minced

1 tsp. crushed red pepper flakes

1 Tbsp. Italian seasoning

½ small yellow onion, minced

....

Method

- Blanche noodles, drain and place in a large bowl.
- Heat the olive oil in a large saucepan over medium-high heat and sauté the onions until they're soft and translucent, about 4-5 minutes. Add the garlic and the anchovies.
- Stir and continue to cook. (The anchovies will literally "melt" into the oil.)
- Add the can of crushed tomatoes (juice and all) along with the tomato paste, Italian seasoning, pepper flakes, and olives.
- Reduce heat and simmer for 20 minutes.
- Pour over pasta and toss to coat with sauce.

Serve immediately.

Note: Not every Paleo pantry list includes tomato paste, so if you're a hard-core Paleo, you can leave it out. The sauce won't be quite as thick, but will taste fine.

tomato-bacon squash pasta (gf/p)

The smoky taste of bacon is sublime when paired with the earthiness of squash and the sweet tomato ties it all together.

Prep Time: 40 m

Serves: 2–4

Calories: 467, Sodium: 803 mg, Dietary Fiber: 7.8 g, Total Fat: 30.6 g, Total Carbs: 31.8 g, Protein: 11.2 g

Ingredients

....

2 cups yellow squash noodles, flat circles cut

1 basket cherry tomatoes, halved

4 strips thick-cut bacon, chopped

1 large red onion, chopped

4 cloves garlic, minced

½ cup white wine

1 ½ cup chicken stock

½ cup fresh arugula, chopped

3 tablespoons olive oil

2 Tbsp. Italian seasoning

....

Method

- In a large skillet, fry the bacon. Remove the bacon and drain off all but a few tablespoons of bacon fat. Add the onion to the pain and cook until it begins to turn golden, then add the garlic and continue to cook.
- Add the white wine. Deglaze the pan (scraping up the caramelized bits with a wooden spoon and stirring them into the sauce).
- Add the chicken stock and the tomatoes. Cook for several minutes until the tomatoes are heated through, then add the Italian seasoning.
- Crumble the bacon back into the pan and add the noodles, stirring to combine everything. Add the arugula and cook another few minutes until the greens wilt.

Serve immediately.

pasta with ricotta & bacon (gf)

You can prepare this pasta and sauce in less time than it takes to have a pizza delivered, and it's a lot better for you!

Prep Time: 55–60 m

Serves: 4

Calories: 353, Sodium: 269 mg, Dietary Fiber: 5.7 g, Total Fat: 7.9 g, Total Carbs: 55.3 g, Protein: 17.4 g

Ingredients

....

4 cups zucchini noodles, flat cut

2 slices bacon, chopped

1 medium yellow onion, diced

1 medium bell pepper, diced

2 large cloves garlic, crushed

1 28-oz. can diced tomatoes

½ cup ricotta cheese

....

Method

- Blanche noodles, drain and place in a large bowl.
- Heat a heavy stockpot over medium heat and fry the bacon until it is beginning to crisp.
- Add the onions and peppers and cook until the onions are translucent, then add the garlic and cook for another minute.
- Add the can of tomatoes, juice and all.
- Simmer for 20 minutes (or longer) to blend flavors.
- Add the cheese to the tomato sauce and stir.
- Add the cooked pasta to the saucepot and stir to blend.

Serve immediately.

Note: If you have some spinach on hand, add about a cup of spinach leaves to give the sauce a little extra fiber.

chili mac (gf)

This quick-fix dinner offers everyone's favorite variation on Mac 'n Cheese with an extra veggie boost.

Prep Time: 25 m

Serves: 4–6

Calories: 398, Sodium: 673 mg, Dietary Fiber: 1.9 g, Total Fat: 21.2 g, Total Carbs: 20.4 g, Protein: 33.6 g

Ingredients

....

2 cups zucchini or yellow squash noodles, flat circles cut

1 pound ground turkey, buffalo, or beef

1 large bell pepper, deseeded and diced

1 package taco seasoning mix

1 14.5-oz. can Mexican-style stewed tomatoes

½ cup water

2 cups shredded Cheddar Cheese (or use "Mexican blend)

....

Method

- Preheat oven to 375.
- In a large skillet brown the meat, onion, and green pepper until the meat is cooked through.
- Add the canned tomatoes (including the juice) the water, and the taco seasoning.
- Simmer 5-10 minutes, stirring occasionally.
- Combine the noodles with the meat/sauce mixture.
- Coat a baking dish with butter or non-stick spray. Place half the noodles in the dish, add half the chili mixture, and to with half the cheese.
- Add another layer of noodles, chili and cheese with the remaining ingredients.
- Bake in the oven for 5 minutes, or until the cheese is melted.

Serve immediately.

CHAPTER 8

DESSERTS

Sometimes all you need at the end of the meal is a piece of sweet, juicy fruit, or a couple of squares of unsweetened dark chocolate. Sometimes, though, you want something a bit more complex, a bit more nuanced. Or let's be honest, you want something that's just…a bit sweeter.

fried apples (gf/v/vg)

This is a Southern specialty that is often served as a side dish with pork or as another Thanksgiving "fixin'. It makes a satisfying dessert for those who can't eat pie. Use a tart apple like Granny Smith for best results.

Prep Time: 20 m

Serves: 4

Calories: 361, Sodium: 0 mg, Dietary Fiber: 3.7 g, Total Fat: 27.4 g, Total Carbs: 34.1 g, Protein: 0.5 g

Ingredients

……………………………………………

4 cups (about 4) peeled or unpeeled apples, flat cut

1/3 cup granulated sugar

½ cup coconut oil

2 ½ Tbsp. cinnamon

……………………………………………

Method
- Melt the coconut oil in a large skillet over medium heat.
- Add the apples.
- Combine the sugar and cinnamon and sprinkle over the apples.
- Cook, stirring occasionally, until apples are tender (5-8 minutes).

Note: Some cooks serve these almost mushy, like warm applesauce, but the dish is also yummy when the apples remain intact with little caramelized edges from the sugar.

gluten-free apple crisp (gf/v)

This delicious dessert is fast and easy to put together and can be served hot or at room temperature. If you're feeling decadent, top with a little ice cream

Prep Time: 70 m

Serves: 6–8

Calories: 191, Sodium: 45 mg, Dietary Fiber: 5.3 g, Total Fat: 8.1 g, Total Carbs: 32.0 g, Protein: 1.7 g

Ingredients

....

6 large apples, unpeeled, cored, flat cut

1/3 cup almond flour

½ cup pecans, chopped

1/3 cup whole oats (not the instant kind)

3 Tbsp. brown sugar

½ stick butter

1 ½ tsp. cinnamon

½ tsp. ginger

Juice of one lemon

....

- Preheat oven to 375 degrees.
- Combine the apples, 1 tsp. cinnamon, ginger, brown sugar and lemon juice. Toss until apple ribbons are coated.
- In a second bowl, combine the almond flour, oats, pecans, brown sugar, and remaining ½ tsp. cinnamon. Use a fork to cut the ingredients together until the texture is crumbly.
- Put the apple mixture into a 10-inch pie pan and cover with the "crisp" topping.
- Bake at 350 for an hour until the filling is piping hot and the topping is crisp and slightly caramelized.
- Remove from oven and let stand for 5 minutes before serving.

apple/rhubarb compote (gf)

This recipe comes in both G and R-rated versions. Serve as is for a homey family dessert, add 1 Tbsp. of Calvados for an adults-only treat.

Prep Time: 40 m

Serves: 6

Calories: 201, Sodium: 30 mg, Dietary Fiber: 5.1 g, Total Fat: 3.9 g, Total Carbs: 43.6 g, Protein: 0.4 g

Ingredients

....

6 Red Delicious Apples, peeled, cored, flat cut

4 rhubarb stalks, cut into one-inch pieces

½ cup granulated sugar

1 Tsp. vanilla extract

2 Tbsp. butter

¼ tsp. ginger

¼ tsp. cinnamon

....

Method

- Combine the butter, sugar, vanilla, spices and (if using) the brandy in a large saucepan. Cook over medium heat until the butter is melted.

- Add the apple ribbons and rhubarb pieces. Simmer for another 15-25 minutes until the fruit is soft and the sauce has thickened. May be served hot or cold.

Note: If rhubarb isn't in season, you can substitute 2 Bartlett pears peeled, cored and cut into bite-sized pieces. Increase the ginger to 1 teaspoon.

sweet potato pudding (gf/v)

This is a spectacularly satisfying gluten-free dessert for a holiday feast. Substitute coconut oil for the butter and almond milk for the milk and it's suitable for vegans.

Prep Time: 75 m

Serves: 6–8

Calories: 335, Sodium: 204 mg, Dietary Fiber: 3.7 g, Total Fat: 11.3 g, Total Carbs: 53.7 g, Protein: 8.2 g

Ingredients

....

1 pound uncooked sweet potatoes, julienned or flat cut

3 eggs, beaten

2 Tbsp. melted butter

2 cups milk (may use low- or non-fat)

½ cup raisins, plumped in ½ hot water and drained

¾ cup pecan halves

1/2 cup dark maple syrup

3 tsp. pumpkin spice mix

2 tablespoons butter, melted

2 cups milk

1 teaspoon cinnamon

....

Method
- Preheat oven to 325 F.
- Coat an 8 x 8 baking pan with butter or non-stick cooking spray.
- Combine all ingredients and pour into prepared pan.

- Bake for an hour.

Note: This can also be made with squash or pumpkin.

Eggs in Pepper Squash

Ingredients		2 Tbsp olive oil	
1 squash	pepper		sea salt
4	eggs	hot sauce for serving	
2 slices bacon			

Procedure

Preheat the oven to 425 degrees F.

Cut the pepper squash into four 3/4"-thick rounds. Scoop the seeds and innards out of each round and discard. Lightly coat both sides of each round with olive oil and place on a lightly-oiled baking sheet. Sprinkle with salt and pepper and bake for 15 minutes, or until tender when poked with a fork.

Remove squash from oven and lower the oven temperature to 350 degrees F.

Crack one egg into one of the squash rounds. Repeat with the remaining 3 eggs.

Place in the oven and bake for 15 minutes.

Serve with cooked crumbled bacon, hot sauce, and any additional toppings you desire.

Servings: 4

Total Time: 40 minutes

Nutrition Facts

Serving size: 1/4 of a recipe (6,2 ounces).

Amount Per Serving		
Calories		201,62
Calories From Fat (60%)		120,87
		% Daily Value
Total Fat 13,42g		21%
Saturated Fat 4,43g		22%
Cholesterol 198,92mg		66%
Sodium 232,5mg		10%
Potassium 482,41mg		14%
Total Carbohydrates 11,71g		4%
Fiber 1,62g		6%
Sugar 0,19g		
Protein 9,35g		19%

Coconut and Chia Seeds Cream

Ingredients

1   can coconut milk

2   Tbsp   Lucuma powder

2   sheets of unflavored gelatin

3   Tbsp   chia seeds

Procedure

In a saucepan over low heat add the coconut milk and dissolve the lucuma powder. Cut the gelatin into pieces and add it to the milk. Stir until dissolved completely. Add chia seeds and stir occasionally until mixture thickens, about 15 minutes. Pour the mixture into individual containers and allow cool before putting them in the refrigerator for at least 2 hours before serving. This breakfast is much more delicious after 24 hours in the refrigerator. Enjoy!

Servings: 4

Total Time: 20 minutes

Nutrition Facts

Serving size: 1/4 of a recipe (2,3 ounces).

Amount Per Serving	
Calories	151,83
Calories From Fat (79%)	120,34
	% Daily Value
Total Fat 14,4g	22%
Saturated Fat 11,27g	56%
Cholesterol 0mg	0%
Sodium 8,39mg	<1%
Potassium 149,2mg	4%
Total Carbohydrates 6,09g	2%
Fiber 2,36g	9%
Protein 1,94g	4%

Paleo Dried Fruit Energy Bars

Ingredients

1 cup dried fruit

1 cup pitted raisins

1 cup dried apricots

3 Tbsp lemon juice

1 handful of chia seeds

Procedure

In a mixer, add the dried fruit and blend until minced well. After checking that it has been minced into tiny pieces (not completely ground), add the raisins and apricots along with two tablespoons of lemon juice. When a batter is formed with all ingredients, remove the mixture from the blender. Format the mass and cut into bars.

Servings: 2

Total Time: 10 minutes

Nutrition Facts

Serving size: 1/2 of a recipe (7,8 ounces).

Amount Per Serving		
Calories		529,86
Calories From Fat (2%)		8,46
		% Daily Value
Total Fat 1,01g		2%
Saturated Fat 0,09g		<1%
Cholesterol 0mg		0%
Sodium 24,8mg		1%
Potassium 1794,79mg		51%
Total Carbohydrates 139,65g		47%
Fiber 11,77g		47%
Sugar 84,14g		
Protein 6,05g		12%

Paleo Pumpkin Pie Smoothie

Ingredients

1 ½ cup milk

2/3 cup pumpkin puree

1/8 cup preferred yogurt

1 banana, peeled

1 cup carrots

2 Tbsp coconut butter

1 Tbsp gelatin

2 tsp vanilla extract

¼ tsp cinnamon

Ice cubes (optional)

Procedure

Place all ingredients in a high powered blender and blend until smooth. Just drink and enjoy!!

Servings: 2

Total Time: 5 minutes

Nutrition Facts

Serving size: 1/2 of a recipe (12,9 ounces).

Amount Per Serving	
Calories	233,92
Calories From Fat (28%)	65,03
	% Daily Value
Total Fat 7,31g	**11%**
Saturated Fat 3,15g	**16%**
Cholesterol 0mg	**0%**
Sodium 197,16mg	**8%**
Potassium 745,08mg	**21%**
Total Carbohydrates 34,45g	**11%**
Fiber 5,17g	**21%**
Sugar 19,12g	
Protein 7,53g	**15%**

Paleo-style Protein Shake

Ingredients	1	banana
1 cup coconut milk	2	Tbsp gelatin powder
½ cup almond milk	4	ice cubes (optional)
2 Tbsp almond butter	1	tsp maple syrup
1 ½ Tbsp cocoa powder		

Procedure

Place all ingredients in a high-powered blender. Blend it for 30 seconds to 1 minute (depending on the power of the blender), or until blended smooth. Serve.

Servings: 2

Total Time: 10 minutes

Nutrition Facts

Serving size: 1/2 of a recipe (9,3 ounces).

Amount Per Serving	
Calories	444,53
Calories From Fat (68%)	300,07
	% Daily Value
Total Fat 35,81g	55%
Saturated Fat 23,96g	120%
Cholesterol 4,88mg	2%
Sodium 79,13mg	3%
Potassium 763,56mg	22%
Total Carbohydrates 31,6g	11%
Fiber 4,63g	19%
Sugar 13,96g	
Protein 8,79g	18%

Paleo-style Salted Cupcakes

Ingredients	2 dried red peppers
6 Tbsp buckwheat flour	4 leaves basil
1 Tbsp olive oil	2 tsp baking powder
3 eggs	2 Tbsp coconut milk
½ tsp salt	

Procedure

Preheat oven to 380° F.

In a deep bowl, add the eggs, coconut milk or cream, basil and peppers and beat. In another bowl add the buckwheat flour with yeast and salt, mix a couple of times to mix well. Add the contents of the second bowl to the first bowl, stirring constantly to air the batter. The texture should be sponge-like. Then, put the paper molds into the individual foil or silicone molds so that they don't break with the weight of the dough. Do not fill the molds to the top - leave a centimeter for it to rise. Bake for 15 minutes. Finally take them out of the pan and let stand on a tray.

Servings: 6

Total Time: 30 minutes

Nutrition Facts

Serving size: 1/6 of a recipe (3,7 ounces).

Amount Per Serving	
Calories	155,54
Calories From Fat (37%)	57,52
	% Daily Value
Total Fat 6,55g	10%
Saturated Fat 2,23g	11%
Cholesterol 93mg	31%
Sodium 398,88mg	17%
Potassium 342,84mg	10%
Total Carbohydrates 19,35g	6%
Fiber 4,15g	17%
Sugar 2,7g	
Protein 6,91g	14%

Paleo-Style Zucchini Bread

Ingredients	2	eggs
1 cup grated zucchini	½	tsp vanilla extract
1 ½ cups almond flour	1	pinch of salt
	2	Tbsp coconut oil
1 tsp baking soda	¼	cup walnuts, chopped
⅓ cup maple syrup or honey		
1 Tbsp cinnamon		

Procedure

Preheat oven to 360F degrees.

Place the eggs, vanilla, coconut oil and maple syrup in a blender and mix until combined well. Add the almond flour, baking soda, salt and ground cinnamon and mix again. Add in the zucchini and walnuts and mix again until smooth. Grease a loaf pan with coconut oil and place the mixture in it. Bake for 35 minutes. Let cool and then remove the bread from the pan.

Servings: 8

Total Time: 45 minutes

Nutrition Facts

Serving size: 1/8 of a recipe (2,6 ounces).

Amount Per Serving	
Calories	196,33
Calories From Fat (32%)	62,47
	% Daily Value
Total Fat 7,27g	11%
Saturated Fat 3,61g	18%
Cholesterol 46,5mg	16%
Sodium 214,88mg	9%
Potassium 131,33mg	4%
Total Carbohydrates 28,58g	10%
Fiber 1,55g	6%
Sugar 8,58g	
Protein 4,78g	10%

Petite Paleo Eggplant Pizzas

Ingredients	Ground black pepper		
For Pizzas	oregano		
2 eggplants	For tomato sauce		
6 slices prosciutto	2	ripe tomatoes	
	1	shallot	
3 Tbsp olive oil	1	dried tomato	
1 cup mushrooms	(optional)		

Procedure

Preheat oven to 360 ° F.

Cut the eggplant into slices. Line the baking pan with foil. Put the eggplant slices on the pan, season with pepper and soak with olive oil. Put the pan in the oven until the eggplant begins to brown. Take the baking pan and to each slice of eggplant, add a tablespoon of tomato sauce, prosciutto slices and the mushrooms. Put the pan back in the oven for about 20-30 minutes.

Tomato sauce

Cut the tomatoes into cubes and chop the shallot. Place in a pan over low heat and cover. Stir occasionally with a spatula, until the tomato is soft enough to cut through with the spatula. Add the dried tomatoes and cover the pan for about 5 minutes, until softened. Remove the pan from heat and in a suitable container, beat until a smooth sauce is achieved.

Servings: 3

Total Time: 55 minutes

Nutrition Facts

Serving size: 1/3 of a recipe (26,4 ounces).

Amount Per Serving	
Calories	266,33
Calories From Fat (11%)	29,45
	% Daily Value
Total Fat 3,28g	5%
Saturated Fat 0,89g	4%
Cholesterol 17,5mg	6%
Sodium 918,23mg	38%
Potassium 1874,43mg	54%
Total Carbohydrates 50,29g	17%
Fiber 13,31g	53%
Sugar 13,8g	
Protein 16,34g	33%

Snowhite Egg Omelette

Ingredients

3 egg whites

1 onion, chopped

1   yellow pepper

1 cup mushrooms, chopped

grated tofu cheese

1 tsp olive oil

Procedure

Chop the onion and green pepper. In a nonstick skillet, sauté the yellow pepper, onion and mushrooms in olive oil until tender. In a meanwhile, in a bowl whisk the egg whites. Add the egg whites to the sautéed vegetables and cook until set. Flip and cook until they have completely set. Add cheese, fold the omelet and place on a plate. Serve hot.

Servings: 2

Total Time: 15 minutes

Nutrition Facts

Serving size: 1/2 of a recipe (8,8 ounces).

Amount Per Serving	
Calories	114,19
Calories From Fat (27%)	31,11
	% Daily Value
Total Fat 3,59g	6%
Saturated Fat 0,46g	2%
Cholesterol 0mg	0%
Sodium 90,71mg	4%
Potassium 497,2mg	14%
Total Carbohydrates 12,53g	4%
Fiber 2,23g	9%
Sugar 3,97g	
Protein 9,83g	20%

Vegetable Soufflé

Ingredients

2 sausages

¼ cup sweet pepper, green pepper, red pepper, paprika

¼ cup grated carrot

½ cup fresh spinach

1 medium onion

3 Tbsp fresh basil

½ tsp sea salt

¼ tsp ground pepper

8 eggs

Procedure

Preheat oven to 380F.

Remove the skin from the sausages and cook them in a pan with onions and a little bit of coconut oil. Undo the sausages with a spoon in order to reduce its size to small crumbs. Remove from heat, place in a container, and let cool. Once the sausages have cooled sufficiently, add the pepper, carrots, spinach and basil. In another bowl, beat the eggs manually with salt and pepper. Combine eggs with sausage and vegetable mixture. You can place the mixture into a rectangular pan but, you could also put ¼ cup of the mixture into individual cupcakes pans. Bake 20 minutes. Serve hot.

Servings: 8

Total Time: 30 minutes

Nutrition Facts

Serving size: 1/8 of a recipe (3,4 ounces).

Avocado and Tuna Tapas

Ingredients

12 ounces in water, drained

1 Tbsp applesauce

3 green onions, sliced

1 red bell pepper, chopped

1 Tbsp balsamic vinegar

black pepper to taste

1 pinch garlic salt, or to taste

2 ripe avocados

Procedure

Stir together tuna, mayonnaise, green onions, red pepper, and balsamic vinegar in a bowl. Season with pepper and garlic salt, then pack the avocado halves with the tuna mixture. Garnish with reserved green onions and a dash of black pepper before serving.

Servings: 4

Total Time: 20 minutes

Nutrition Facts

Serving size: 1/4 of a recipe (14 ounces).

Amount Per Serving	
Calories	504,33
Calories From Fat (38%)	192,37
	% Daily Value
Total Fat 22,27g	34%
Saturated Fat 4,05g	20%
Cholesterol 108,06mg	36%
Sodium 1062,76mg	44%
Potassium 1159,27mg	33%
Total Carbohydrates 12,24g	4%
Fiber 7,03g	28%
Sugar 2,89g	
Protein 62,57g	125%

Bacon Caprese Salad

Ingredients

4 slices bacon, diced

½ cup chopped celery

½ cup honey

½ cup apple vinegar

½ cup sliced shallots

¼ cup roasted garlic

2 Tbsp lemon juice

½ Tbsp applesauce

4 Tbsp canola oil

Kosher salt

ground black pepper

For salad:

¾ lb tofu cheese, thinly sliced

2 tomatoes

1 Tbsp marjoram leaves

Procedure

Make the vinaigrette: In a large food processor, process ½ lb. bacon (reserve fat), celery, honey, vinegar, shallots, garlic, lemon juice, and applesauce until smooth. With the processor running, slowly add oil and the reserved bacon fat; season with salt and pepper.

Make the salad: Combine tofu cheese, tomatoes, and marjoram; season with salt and pepper and drizzle with vinaigrette. Garnish with some bacon.

Servings: 6

Degree of Difficulty: Easy

Total Time: 15 minutes

Nutrition Facts

Serving size: 1/6 of a recipe (6,7 ounces).

Amount Per Serving	
Calories	352,24
Calories From Fat (60%)	209,73
	% Daily Value
Total Fat 23,67g	36%
Saturated Fat 4,91g	25%
Cholesterol 17,61mg	6%
Sodium 277,09mg	12%
Potassium 367,45mg	10%
Total Carbohydrates 37,03g	12%
Fiber 1,19g	5%
Sugar 23,68g	
Protein 9,07g	18%

Ground Beef with Swiss Chard

Ingredients	½ tsp	garlic powder
¾ lbs chopped beef	1 tsp	ground pepper
2 cups Swiss chard	½ tsp	ground cumin
¼ cup cashews	1 tsp	oregano
1 Tbsp coconut oil	Himalayan salt	

Procedure

In a saucepan, melt the coconut oil and cook the meat over medium heat. Add the cumin, oregano, garlic powder, ground pepper and salt. Mix well. Add the chopped Swiss chard leaves and cook for 5 minutes more. Remove from heat and add the cashews. Serve.

Servings: 4

Total Time: 40 minutes

Nutrition Facts

Serving size: 1/4 of a recipe (3,9 ounces).

Amount Per Serving	
Calories	269,68
Calories From Fat (74%)	198,26
	% Daily Value
Total Fat 21,73g	33%
Saturated Fat 10,14g	51%
Cholesterol 63,79mg	21%
Sodium 98,07mg	4%
Potassium 320,57mg	9%
Total Carbohydrates 2,09g	<1%
Fiber 0,69g	3%
Sugar 0,32g	
Protein 15,83g	32%

Grilled Salmon with Saffron & Olives

Ingredients

1 cup plum tomatoes

½ cup black olives

4 Tbsp virgin olive oil

4 cloves fresh garlic

½ tsp fresh thyme

½ tsp kosher salt

Saffron,

(15 to 20 threads)

ground black pepper

4 salmon fillets

Procedure

Heat a gas grill or charcoal grill.

In a medium bowl, combine the tomatoes, olives, olive oil, garlic, thyme, salt, saffron, and pepper to taste.

Set one piece of salmon and sprinkle lightly with salt and pepper. Spoon a quarter of the tomato mixture over the fish and seal tightly. Repeat to make four packets.

Place on the grill and cook with the grill covered about 8-10 minutes. Let the salmon rest for a few minutes before serving.

Servings: 4

Total Time: 25 minutes

Nutrition Facts

Serving size: 1/4 of a recipe (8.7 ounces).

Amount Per Serving	
Calories	332,52
Calories From Fat (58%)	193,27
	% Daily Value
Total Fat 21,75g	33%
Saturated Fat 3,56g	18%
Cholesterol 39,12mg	13%
Sodium 3475,89mg	145%
Potassium 312,27mg	9%
Total Carbohydrates 1,53g	<1%
Fiber 0,39g	2%
Sugar 0,03g	
Protein 31,34g	63%

Mottled Pomegranate & Orange Salad

Ingredients

For the salad:

2 cup lettuce, chopped

1 avocado

½ mango, diced

1 orange

¾ cup almonds

For the vinaigrette:

4 Tbsp olive oil

2 Tbsp balsamic vinegar

3 Tbsp pomegranate juice

Salt and black pepper

Procedure

In a deep salad bowl, chop the lettuce, and add the chopped, avocado, orange, the pomegranate and whole almonds.

For the vinaigrette: In a bowl, mix olive oil, vinegar, pomegranate juice, salt and black pepper. Mix to combine well. Pour the vinaigrette over the salad and serve.

Servings: 6

Total Time: 20 minutes

Nutrition Facts

Serving size: 1/6 of a recipe (9.2 ounces).

Amount Per Serving	
Calories	270,4
Calories From Fat (36%)	97,81
	% Daily Value
Total Fat 11,42g	18%
Saturated Fat 1,49g	7%
Cholesterol 0mg	0%
Sodium 15,14mg	<1%
Potassium 675,61mg	19%
Total Carbohydrates 43,48g	14%
Fiber 10,38g	42%
Sugar 30,26g	
Protein 4,11g	8%

Mussels with Tarragon & Apple Vinaigrette

Ingredients

2 lb   mussels

1/3   cup applesauce

2 hard-boiled eggs

2 Tbsp apple vinegar

¼ tsp salt

¼ tsp black pepper

1/4   cup olive oil

½ cup celery, chopped

½ cup sour onions

¼ cup fresh tarragon

Procedure

Cook mussels with water and applesauce in a pot over moderately high heat, covered, until mussels just open wide, checking frequently after 4 minutes and transferring opened mussels to a large bowl using a slotted spoon. (Discard any unopened mussels after 10 minutes.)

Pour cooking liquid through a fine-mesh sieve into a 1- to 2-quart heavy saucepan and boil until reduced to about 3 tablespoons, about 5 minutes. Transfer to a bowl.

Finely chop eggs, then add to reduced liquid along with vinegar, salt, and pepper. Add oil in a slow stream, whisking, then whisk in celery, onions, and tarragon. Season the vinaigrette with salt and pepper.

Remove mussels from shells and reserve 1 half shell from each mussel. Stir mussels into vinaigrette and marinate, covered and chilled, at least 1 hour. Rinse and dry reserved mussel shells, then chill in a sealed plastic bag until ready to use.

Arrange shells on a large platter lined with seaweed and spoon a mussel with some vinaigrette into each.

Servings: 8

Total Time: 1 hour and 45 minutes

Nutrition Facts

Serving size: 1/8 of a recipe (6 ounces).

Amount Per Serving	
Calories	192,29
Calories From Fat (50%)	96,5
	% Daily Value
Total Fat 10,84g	17%
Saturated Fat 1,89g	9%
Cholesterol 84,79mg	28%
Sodium 473,34mg	20%
Potassium 432,05mg	12%
Total Carbohydrates 5,72g	2%
Fiber 0,32g	1%
Sugar 0,7g	
Protein 15,5g	31%

Purslane with Pork & Green Tomatoes

Ingredients	4,5	lbs purslane

¾ lb pork, chopped

½ kg green tomatoes

1 onion

6 serrano chilies green

4 cloves garlic

2 Tbsp oil

1 bay leaf

½ cup cilantro leaves

Salt to taste

Vegetable bouillon powdered, to taste

Procedure

Place the pork, onion, clove garlic and 1 bay leaf in a pot, cover with water and add salt to taste. Let boil over high heat, reduce the flame, cover and simmer until tender. Meanwhile, wash the purslane and separate the leaves from the stems. Steam the leaves in a large pot with water and salt. Then drain well. On the side, boil the tomatoes together with serrano peppers in a pan with water until tender, but before falling apart. Heat the oil in a saucepan over low heat. Mix the cooked tomatoes and peppers with 2 cloves of garlic, cilantro and 2 cups of meat broth. Pour into the pan with the hot oil, cover and cook for 10 minutes. Add the meat, purslane and bouillon powder; let everything simmer together for a few minutes. Serve warm.

Servings: 6

Total Time: 30 minutes

Nutrition Facts

Serving size: 1/6 of a recipe (15.9 ounces).

Amount Per Serving	
Calories	369,51
Calories From Fat (72%)	267,02
	% Daily Value
Total Fat 29,75g	46%
Saturated Fat 8,88g	44%
Cholesterol 37,28mg	12%
Sodium 726,54mg	30%
Potassium 1895,65mg	54%
Total Carbohydrates 17,04g	6%
Fiber 0,81g	3%
Sugar 1,22g	
Protein 11,7g	23%

Spanish Paleo Lobster Stew

Ingredients

3	Tbsp coconut butter	1 liter water
2	onions	1 white pepper
5	garlic cloves	¼ cup pine nuts
1	ripe tomato	salt
2	lobsters	

Procedure

In an earthenware dish, gently fry the finely-chopped onions with 3 of the garlic cloves, also finely chopped, and the peeled and chopped tomato. Cut the lobster into thick slices. Set aside the coral and roe, if any. Add the lobster flesh to the vegetable mixture, brown and add most of the stock. Bring to the boil and season with salt and pepper.

In a mortar (or blender), crush the remaining garlic clove, the coral and roe from the lobster and the pine nuts. Dilute with a little stock and add to the lobster and vegetables. Cook for a further 10 minutes.

Servings: 4

Total Time: 1 hour and 30 minutes

Nutrition Facts

Serving size: 1/4 of a recipe (23.5 ounces).

Amount Per Serving	
Calories	375,35
Calories From Fat (37%)	138,44
	% Daily Value
Total Fat 15,8g	24%
Saturated Fat 2,26g	11%
Cholesterol 290,5mg	97%
Sodium 1581,53mg	66%
Potassium 1167,59mg	33%
Total Carbohydrates 12,34g	4%
Fiber 2,56g	10%
Sugar 5,59g	
Protein 45,82g	92%

Tenderloin with Fine Herbs Stew

Ingredients

1 ½ lbs pork loin

2 cups vegetable broth

4 cloves garlic

½ cup applesauce

4 Tbsp olive oil

Herbs: bay leaf

thyme, rosemary

Procedure

In a large pot, on medium high heat, pour enough oil to cover the bottom with a thin film. Add the garlic cloves, halved and enough herbs enough to cover the bottom of the pot. When the oil is hot cook the tenderloin about 5 minutes per side. Place it on top of the garlic and herbs.

After that time has elapsed, remove the meat and add the applesauce while scraping any herbs that may have stuck to the bottom of the pan. Boil everything about 2-3 minutes. Add the vegetable broth. Lower the heat to medium / low and out the meat back in the pot. Boil for an hour and a half. After time has elapsed, careful not to burn yourself, cut into slices and put it back in the pan, heating over low heat another 20 minutes.

Servings: 6

Total Time: 1 hour and 5 minutes

Nutrition Facts

Serving size: 1/6 of a recipe (8 ounces).

Amount Per Serving	
Calories	289,22
Calories From Fat (44%)	126,33
	% Daily Value
Total Fat 14,19g	22%
Saturated Fat 2,91g	15%
Cholesterol 75,66mg	25%
Sodium 598,51mg	25%
Potassium 590,75mg	17%
Total Carbohydrates 11,73g	4%
Fiber 1,33g	5%
Sugar 1,93g	
Protein 27,56g	55%

Watermelon Raw Vegetables Soup

Ingredients

14 oz   tomatoes

1 ½ cup watermelon   pepper

1 can   tomato
juice

1 tsp   parsley,
fresh

3 Tbsp lime juice

¼ tsp salt

Garnish:

lime, cilantro

Procedure

Combine all ingredients in a food processor and blend until smooth. If you prefer gazpacho chunky, pulse the mixture into smaller chunks.

Sprinkle with the salt and the pepper to a taste. Garnish with cilantro and lime wedges.

Servings: 2

Total Time: 10 minutes

Nutrition Facts

Serving size: 1/2 of a recipe (15.8 ounces).

Amount Per Serving	
Calories	112,13
Calories From Fat (6%)	6,27
	% Daily Value
Total Fat 0,77g	1%
Saturated Fat 0,11g	<1%
Cholesterol 0mg	0%
Sodium 585,26mg	24%
Potassium 933,12mg	27%
Total Carbohydrates 28,47g	9%
Fiber 5,66g	23%
Sugar 15,98g	
Protein 3,46g	7%

Broiled Chicken with Tomato Sauce

Ingredients

Cooking spray

3   lbs chicken, cut

1   Tbsp   olive oil

1   onion, chopped

2   Tbsp   tapioca flour or buckwheat

1 ½ cups broth

3 Tbsp tomato paste

1 tsp   maple syrup

1 tsp   dry mustard

Procedure

Heat broiler or grill. Spray rack. Spray chicken pieces. Broil 30 minutes, turning often, and spraying again at each turn.

Heat butter in saucepan. Add onion and sauté until limp. Sprinkle with flour and cook, stirring, 2 to 3 minutes. Remove from heat and add boiling broth, beating vigorously with wire whisk to prevent lumping. Return to heat and cook, stirring, until smooth and thick.

Stir in tomato paste, maple sauce, and mustard. Serve over broiled chicken.

Servings: 4

Total Time: 50 minutes

Nutrition Facts

Serving size: 1/4 of a recipe.

Amount Per Serving	
Calories	311
Calories From Fat (38%)	119,3
	% Daily Value
Total Fat 13g	20%
Saturated Fat 4g	20%
Cholesterol 116mg	39%
Sodium 189mg	8%
Total Carbohydrates 10g	3%
Fiber 1g	4%
Protein 37g	74%

Grilled Sour Goat with Garlic

Ingredients

4,4 lbs goat	1 tsp ground chili
8 garlic cloves	¼ cup white vinegar
2 tsp ground cumin	¼ cup olive oil
2 tsp sweet paprika	1 lemon, juiced
	3 tsp dried oregano

Procedure

In a mortar with the pestle, beat garlic with 2 tablespoon salt. Place in a large bowl with remaining ingredients and toss goat to coat in marinade. Cover with plastic wrap and refrigerate for 2 hours or preferably overnight. Remove from fridge 1 hour before cooking.

Cook goat, basting occasionally with remaining marinade, over a medium fire or coals for 45 minutes for medium or until cooked to your liking.

Servings: 6

Total Time: 1 hour and 50 minutes

Nutrition Facts

Serving size: 1/6 of a recipe (13 ounces).

Amount Per Serving	
Calories	458,2
Calories From Fat (33%)	152,23
	% Daily Value
Total Fat 17,06g	26%
Saturated Fat 3,66g	18%
Cholesterol 190mg	63%
Sodium 275,76mg	11%
Potassium 1341,72mg	38%
Total Carbohydrates 3,43g	1%
Fiber 0,51g	2%
Sugar 0,33g	
Protein 69,15g	138%

Jalapeño Tuna with Tomato Burgers

Ingredients

1 cup of tuna

1 Jalapeño pepper

3 Tbsp tomato paste

1 egg

1 red onion, chopped

2 clove garlic

1 Tbsp coconut flour

Salt and pepper to taste

Decoration

Lettuce, Basil

Procedure

Preheat oven to 350'F.

In a medium bowl, place all burger ingredients and stir until well combined. Using your hands, carefully roll and flatten your tuna mixture into 6, even sized burger patties. Line a baking tray with baking/parchment paper and set aside. Place burger patties in a baking tray and cook for 5-10 minutes, until set and cooked through. Serve hot.

You can decorate the plate with lettuce leafs, put the tuna burger and then sprinkle over some fresh basil and a few extra slices of chili.

Servings: 6

Total Time: 20 minutes

Nutrition Facts

Serving size: 1/6 of a recipe (2.2 ounces).

Amount Per Serving	
Calories	106,13
Calories From Fat (41%)	43,1
	% Daily Value
Total Fat 4,86g	7%
Saturated Fat 1,52g	8%
Cholesterol 43,04mg	14%
Sodium 231,83mg	10%
Potassium 193,77mg	6%
Total Carbohydrates 6,7g	2%
Fiber 0,6g	2%
Sugar 1,2g	
Protein 8,91g	18%

Lemony Grilled Chicken Liver

Ingredients	4	Tbsp coconut oil
1 lb chicken livers, trimmed	2	lemon juice
2 Tbsp olive oil	4 minced	sprigs Italian parsley,
Salt		
Pepper		

Procedure

Light the grill and let the coals or wood get very hot. Soak four 6- to 8-inch/15- to 20-centimeter wooden skewers in water for 30 minutes.

Divide the livers equally among the 4 skewers, then brush them with the oil and season them generously with salt and pepper.

Grill the livers, until well browned and cooked through, 2 to 3 minutes per side.

Meanwhile, in a saucepan melt the butter and mix in the lemon juice and parsley. When the livers are cooked, brush the lemon sauce over them thoroughly. Serve hot.

Servings: 4

Total Time: 25 minutes

Nutrition Facts

Serving size: 1/4 of a recipe (5.3 ounces).

Amount Per Serving	
Calories	300,18
Calories From Fat (70%)	210,84
	% Daily Value
Total Fat 23,79g	37%
Saturated Fat 10,01g	50%
Cholesterol 421,76mg	141%
Sodium 155,07mg	6%
Potassium 282,19mg	8%
Total Carbohydrates 1,98g	<1%
Fiber 0,09g	<1%
Sugar 0,38g	
Protein 19,38g	39%

Marinated White Fish with Mango

Ingredients

2,20 lbs white fish

2 mangoes, cubed

4 tomatoes, chopped

1 avocado, cubed

1 Tbsp olive oil

2/3 cup lemon juice

½ orange juice

1 serrano pepper, chopped

1 cup spring onions, thinly sliced

¼ cup cilantro

Salt and pepper, to taste

Procedure

Place fish, lemon juice, orange juice, olive oil and pepper in a glass or plastic container. Mix well, cover and refrigerate for 2 hours. When the fish is ready, add the onion and mango. Set aside for 15 minutes. Remove fish from refrigerator; carefully wrap the tomatoes and cilantro and season with salt and pepper.

Servings: 6

Total Time: 1 hour and 20 minutes

Nutrition Facts

Serving size: 1/6 of a recipe (13.7 ounces).

Amount Per Serving	
Calories	134,76
Calories From Fat (46%)	61,43

	% Daily Value
Total Fat 7,21g	11%
Saturated Fat 1g	5%
Cholesterol 0mg	0%
Sodium 438,93mg	18%
Potassium 815,85mg	23%
Total Carbohydrates 18,58g	6%
Fiber 5,61g	22%
Sugar 9g	
Protein 3,43g	7%

Orange, Watercress and Fennel Salad

Ingredients

1	orange, grated	1 cup watercress
1	fennel bulb	1 Tbsp apple cider
1	pear	3 Tbsp virgin olive oil
		¼ tsp salt
		tofu cheese (optional)

Procedure

In a salad bowl place the orange juice, zest, apple cider vinegar, oil and salt. Beat with a whisk or fork until all ingredients are fully combined. Make sure it is seasoned to taste.

Chop the fennel bulb. Set aside. Remove the pear core, divide it into quarters, and slice into thin slices, again with the help of a mandolin or knife. Add the fennel and pear slices to the bowl with the dressing and mix well. Let marinate for at least 20 minutes. Just before serving the salad, add the watercress, the set aside fennel leaves and tofu cheese (if desired) and mix. Serve.

Servings: 4

Total Time: 35 minutes

Nutrition Facts

Serving size: 1/4 of a recipe (5.5 ounces).

Amount Per Serving	
Calories	149,34
Calories From Fat (61%)	91,45
	% Daily Value
Total Fat 10,36g	16%
Saturated Fat 1,41g	7%
Cholesterol 0mg	0%
Sodium 180,37mg	8%
Potassium 378,24mg	11%
Total Carbohydrates 14,72g	5%
Fiber 3,52g	14%
Sugar 6,96g	
Protein 1,27g	3%

Paleo Butternut Squash Soup

Ingredients

3 lbs squash, cut into ½-inch chunks

1 cup red onion, sliced

2 cup vegetable broth

1 cup coconut milk

2 tsp olive oil

4 cloves garlic, minced

1 bay leaf

½ tsp salt

Procedure

Preheat oven to 450° F.

Place the squash and onion with half oil and salt on a rimmed baking sheet. Roast in a single layer until browned and soft, about 25-30 minutes.

Transfer the vegetables to a large saucepan with the remaining 1 teaspoon oil and cook over medium-low heat, stirring often, for 3-5 minutes. Add garlic and cook for another 30 seconds. Add the broths, bay leaf and coconut milk; bring to a boil. Reduce heat to medium-low, cover and simmer for 10 minutes more.

At the end, remove bay leaf and transfer squash mixture to a blender. Puree until smooth. Serve.

Servings: 6

Total Time: 55 minutes

Nutrition Facts

Serving size: 1/6 of a recipe (12.7 ounces).

Amount Per Serving	
Calories	285,85
Calories From Fat (40%)	114,95
	% Daily Value
Total Fat 13,47g	21%
Saturated Fat 8,62g	43%
Cholesterol 0,82mg	<1%
Sodium 780,06mg	33%
Potassium 1038,38mg	30%
Total Carbohydrates 41,25g	14%
Fiber 5,75g	23%
Sugar 5,01g	
Protein 5,45g	11%

Paleo Glazed Salmon Fillets

Ingredients

2 lbs salmon filets

1 Tbsp oregano, chopped

1/3   cup apple vinegar

5 cloves garlic, chopped

1 Tbsp white wine

1 Tbsp honey

4 tsp mustard

Salt and pepper

Procedure

Preheat oven to 400 °F.

Spray a small saucepan with cooking spray. Add the garlic and sauté over medium heat, stirring constantly, until smooth, about 3 minutes. Stir in the white wine, honey, balsamic vinegar, mustard, salt and pepper. Cook, uncovered, for 3 minutes or until slightly thickened.

Line a baking pan with foil and spray with cooking spray. Arrange the salmon filets in the baking pan. Glaze with balsamic vinegar mixture and sprinkle with oregano. Bake 10 to 15 minutes or until fish flakes easily with a fork. Use a spatula to move the steaks to a platter, leaving the skin on the tray. Serve hot.

Servings: 4

Total Time: 30 minutes

Nutrition Facts

Serving size: 1/4 of a recipe (9 ounces).

Amount Per Serving	
Calories	832,46
Calories From Fat (28%)	235,4
	% Daily Value
Total Fat 26,21g	40%
Saturated Fat 5,91g	30%
Cholesterol 351,54mg	117%
Sodium 184,47mg	8%
Potassium 2242,14mg	64%
Total Carbohydrates 10,38g	3%
Fiber 0,7g	3%
Sugar 7,61g	
Protein 138,18g	276%

Paleo Shrimp Stuffed Avocados

Ingredients	1	Tbsp onion powder
1 ½ cups shrimps, boiled	1	tsp black pepper
1 Tbsp lemon juice	1	Tbsp paprika
4 avocados, cut in halves	1	tomato

Procedure

With the knife, peel and cut avocado in halves. Place avocados on a plate with the cut sides facing up. In a medium bowl, mix the shrimp, lemon juice, onion powder and pepper. Place shrimp mixture on each avocado, covering them generously. Chop the tomato. Sprinkle the top of each stuffed avocado with paprika and top with tomato before serving.

Servings: 6

Total Time: 15 minutes

Nutrition Facts

Serving size: 1/6 of a recipe
(5   ounces).

Amount Per Serving	
Calories	205,4
Calories From Fat (73%)	150,94
	% Daily Value
Total Fat 18g	28%
Saturated Fat 2,49g	12%
Cholesterol 1,89mg	<1%
Sodium 20,48mg	<1%
Potassium 679,59mg	19%
Total Carbohydrates 12,55g	4%
Fiber 8,69g	35%
Sugar 1,2g	
Protein 2,95g	6%

Paleo Turkey Breast with Garlic Sauce

Ingredients	1 tsp	cumin
1/3 cup parsley	¼ tsp	cayenne pepper
6 garlic cloves, minced	1 ½ lbs turkey breast	
½ cup lemon juice	1 Tbsp olive oil, for brushing	
3 Tbsp olive oil		
1 tsp paprika		

Procedure

In a blender, mix all sauce ingredients together. Set aside.

Broil or grill the turkey breasts brushing with olive oil to keep moist. Grill on each side about 4 minutes.

Top each slice with some of the sauce (to taste). Serve hot.

Servings: 6

Total Time: 25 minutes

Nutrition Facts

Serving size: 1/6 of a recipe.

Amount Per Serving	
Calories	229
Calories From Fat (47%)	108,47
	% Daily Value
Total Fat 12g	18%
Saturated Fat 2g	10%
Cholesterol 75mg	25%
Sodium 52mg	2%
Total Carbohydrates 2g	<1%
Fiber 0g	0%
Protein 28g	56%

Baked Garlicky Carrots with Lemon

Ingredients		1	lemon juice
3 ½ cups carrots, sliced		1	lemon zest
2 onions, cut		4	Tbsp olive oil
5 cloves garlic, pressed		2	tsp cumin
			Ground black pepper

Procedure

Preheat oven to 390F.

In a bowl mix the lemon juice with the cumin, oil and pepper. Pour over sliced carrots, onions and garlic. Mix well and arrange on a tray lined with parchment paper. Bake for 20-25 minutes, occasionally stirring. Serve immediately.

Servings: 4

Nutrition Facts

Serving size: 1/4 of a recipe (3.1 ounces).

Amount Per Serving	
Calories	122
Calories From Fat (76%)	92,31
	% Daily Value
Total Fat 10,46g	16%
Saturated Fat 1,45g	7%
Cholesterol 0mg	0%
Sodium 4,91mg	<1%
Potassium 126,94mg	4%
Total Carbohydrates 7,47g	2%
Fiber 1,36g	5%
Sugar 3,07g	
Protein 0,94g	2%

Eggplant Goofy Snack

Ingredients	2 Tbsp maple syrup
1 lb eggplant	½ cup olive oil
¾ tsp paprika	sea salt
4 Tbsp vine vinegar	

Procedure

Slice eggplant into thin strips, half crosswise.

In a bowl, whisk together oil, maple syrup, paprika and vinegar. Place eggplant strips in the mixture a few at a time, turning to make sure each is completely coated. Marinate about 2 hours. Then, place strips on baking sheets or dehydrator trays or in the oven or, you can dry in a food dehydrator

If you use an oven; sprinkle on a little salt. Place in oven on lowest setting for 10 to 12 hours (ovens' lowest setting varies, thus drying time will vary) or until dry and fairly crisp, turning strips partway through. Check occasionally, and if any oil pools on the sheets, blot with a paper towel.

If you use a food dehydrator, act according to the manufacturer's instruction.

When ready, store strips in an airtight container or plastic bag. Place a paper towel under or around strips to absorb any excess.

Servings: 30

Preparation Time: 30 minutes

Total Time: 24 hours

Nutrition Facts

Serving size: 1/30 of a recipe (0,8 ounces).

Amount Per Serving	
Calories	40,96
Calories From Fat (78%)	32,13
	% Daily Value
Total Fat 3,64g	6%
Saturated Fat 0,5g	3%
Cholesterol 0mg	0%
Sodium 1,06mg	<1%
Potassium 41,34mg	1%
Total Carbohydrates 2,15g	<1%
Fiber 0,53g	2%
Sugar 1,49g	
Protein 0,17g	<1%

Ginger Spiced Butternut Chips

Ingredients

1 ½ cups butternut squash

2 Tbsp coconut oil, melted

1 tsp   ginger

¼ tsp   nutmeg

½   tsp cinnamon

1/8 tsp cloves

Pinch salt

Stevia to taste (optional)

Procedure

Preheat the oven to 250 F.

Clean and peel the butternut squash, and slice thinly on a mandolin. Place the butternut squash a bowl.

In another bowl, mix melted coconut oil, and add in ginger, nutmeg, cinnamon and cloves. If you like more sweet (butternut squash is naturally sweet) sprinkle in a few drops Stevia. Pour the oil mixture over the butternut squash and mix well to allow it everywhere.

Place the slices close to each other on a baking tray lined with parchment paper. Place the baking tray in the oven and cook for about 1.5 hour or until crispy.

Although the chips shouldn't burn at low temperature, you should keep an eye on them. When done, let them cool down and store in an air-tight container for up to a week.

Servings: 4

Total Time: 1 hour and 40 minutes

Nutrition Facts

Serving size: 1/4 of a recipe (2,1 ounces).

Amount Per Serving	
Calories	84,38
Calories From Fat (71%)	59,65
	% Daily Value
Total Fat 6,92g	11%
Saturated Fat 5,93g	30%
Cholesterol 0mg	0%
Sodium 2,38mg	<1%
Potassium 189,48mg	5%
Total Carbohydrates 6,6g	2%
Fiber 1,28g	5%
Sugar 1,21g	
Protein 0,56g	1%

Paleo Citrus Broccoli

Ingredients

4	cups	broccoli
2	Tbsp	olive oil
1	lemon	

2 Tbsp Sesame (optional)

salt & pepper

½ orange

Procedure

Preheat oven to 475 degrees F.

Spread the broccoli florets on a baking sheet and drizzle with olive oil. Gently toss the florets in the oil to coat. Sprinkle with sesame if desired.

Cook in oven for 20 minutes.

Remove from oven and squeeze the lemon and orange juice on top of the broccoli. Place the broccoli back into the oven for 15 more minutes.

Remove the broccoli from the oven and season with salt and pepper.

Serve immediately.

Servings: 6

Total Time: 30 minutes

Nutrition Facts

Serving size: 1/6 of a recipe (9,3 ounces).

Amount Per Serving	
Calories	122,41
Calories From Fat (42%)	50,93
	% Daily Value
Total Fat 5,86g	9%
Saturated Fat 1,04g	5%
Cholesterol 1,47mg	<1%
Sodium 87,61mg	4%
Potassium 791,3mg	23%
Total Carbohydrates 15,93g	5%
Fiber 1,44g	6%
Sugar 0,02g	
Protein 7,79g	16%

Paleo Flourless Chocolate Cake

Ingredients

4   eggs

1   cup   almonds, ground

1 cup cocoa

4 Tbsp coconut butter

¾ cup maple syrup

Procedure

Preheat oven to 350 degrees F.

In a bowl beat eggs yolks until get creamy. In another bowl beat with mixer egg whites well. Unite the yolks mixture with the egg whites mixture. Stir. Add in cocoa, butter and the ground almonds. Stir well for 2-3 minutes. Grease a round baking pan and pour in the batter.

Bake for 30-35 minutes. When ready cool a cake on a wire rack. Before serving pour maple syrup over the top.

Servings: 6

Total Time: 35 minutes

Nutrition Facts

Serving size: 1/6 of a recipe (3,1 ounces).

Amount Per Serving	
Calories	315,54
Calories From Fat (49%)	155,27
	% Daily Value
Total Fat 18,14g	28%
Saturated Fat 4,56g	23%
Cholesterol 124mg	41%
Sodium 55,87mg	2%
Potassium 246,4mg	7%
Total Carbohydrates 32,09g	11%
Fiber 2,51g	10%
Sugar 27,94g	
Protein 9,06g	18%

Paleo Hot Peppers Cups

Ingredients		4	basil leaves fresh
4 eggs		1	Tbsp olive oil
2 tsp	baking powder	8	Tbsp buckwheat flour
3 Tbsp coconut milk			
½ tsp	salt		
3 dried red peppers			

Procedure

Preheat oven to 380F.

In a bowl beat the eggs, coconut milk or cream, basil and hot peppers.

In another bowl mix the buckwheat flour with the baking powder and salt.

Unite the egg mixture with the flour mixture and stir well. The texture should be like a sponge.

Pour the batter in cups (3/4 cup full).

Bake in a oven for 15-20 minutes.

When ready leave to cool on the rack and then unmold. Serve.

Servings: 4

Total Time: 25 minutes

Nutrition Facts

Serving size: 1/4 of a recipe (7,6 ounces).

Amount Per Serving	
Calories	289,23
Calories From Fat (35%)	102,29
	% Daily Value
Total Fat 11,65g	18%
Saturated Fat 4,06g	20%
Cholesterol 186mg	62%
Sodium 615,43mg	26%
Potassium 551,76mg	16%
Total Carbohydrates 36,32g	12%
Fiber 6,29g	25%
Sugar 5,8g	
Protein 12,56g	25%

Paleo Peppermint Green Tea Shake

Ingredients

½ banana (frozen)

¾ cup   spinach

4 mint leaves

1 tangerine

¼ stick of celery

½ cup Green tea

Procedure

In a blender infuse the tea, and put all ingredients. Blend well several seconds and your shake is ready! It's great, super sweet, creamy and refreshing. You can add a few drops of Stevia to taste.

Servings: 2

Total Time: 8 minutes

Nutrition Facts

Serving size: 1/2 of a recipe (6,9 ounces).

Amount Per Serving	
Calories	66,34
Calories From Fat (6%)	3,91
	% Daily Value
Total Fat 0,47g	<1%
Saturated Fat 0,09g	<1%
Cholesterol 0mg	0%
Sodium 46,36mg	2%
Potassium 495,01mg	14%
Total Carbohydrates 15,61g	5%
Fiber 2,97g	12%
Sugar 9,1g	
Protein 2,25g	5%

Paleo Quick Crackers

Ingredients		1	egg
1	cup almond meal	Sesame (optional)	
2	tsp coconut butter	pinch	of salt

Procedure

Preheat your oven to 350 degrees Fahrenheit.

In a blender or food processor add all ingredients (except sesame). Combine well at medium speed. Do not allow the mixture to become sticky.

Roll the mixture into a ball and place between two sheets of baking paper, roll out to your desired thickness.

Remove the top layer of baking paper and place on an oven tray. Sprinkle with sesame if desired. Bake for 20 minutes. Remove from the oven and allow cool prior to cutting into crackers. Enjoy.

Servings: 6

Total Time: 30 minutes

Nutrition Facts

Serving size: 1/6 of a recipe (1,1 ounces).

Amount Per Serving	
Calories	112,12
Calories From Fat (30%)	34,01
	% Daily Value
Total Fat 3,89g	6%
Saturated Fat 1,27g	6%
Cholesterol 34,39mg	11%
Sodium 58,01mg	2%
Potassium 84,55mg	2%
Total Carbohydrates 17,23g	6%
Fiber 1,67g	7%
Sugar 6,5g	
Protein 3,08g	6%

Simple Paleo Pancakes

Ingredients	2	tsp almond flour
1	egg (large)	Cinnamon
1	banana	2 Tbsp coconut oil (or olive oil)

Procedure

In a bowl, beat the egg. Mash the banana with a fork to reach a puree consistency and add the egg. Keep whipping. Add the cinnamon and a teaspoon of the almond flour (ground almonds).

Pour the mixture into a small skillet greased with oil (not too much oil, just enough to prevent sticking). Leave it a few seconds over high heat and then lower to the lowest setting. In a few minutes, when the batter begins to set, turn the heat back up for a couple of seconds, then lower the heat again and leave it for a couple of minutes over low heat.

Serve with maple syrup, honey or your favorite fruits.

Servings: 3

Nutrition Facts

Serving size: 1/3 of a recipe (2,4 ounces).

Amount Per Serving	
Calories	143,31
Calories From Fat (65%)	93,66
	% Daily Value
Total Fat 10,8g	17%
Saturated Fat 8,41g	42%
Cholesterol 62mg	21%
Sodium 24,09mg	1%
Potassium 165,67mg	5%
Total Carbohydrates 10,43g	3%
Fiber 1,07g	4%
Sugar 4,88g	
Protein 2,7g	5%

Sultana Carrot Paleo Cake

Ingredients   ½ cup coconut oil

1 cup coconut flour   ½ cup honey

4 eggs   2 tsp cinnamon

½ cup hazelnut flour   1 tsp vinegar

2 cups carrot grated   ½ tsp baking soda

½ cup sultana, seedless   ½ tsp salt

Procedure

Preheat oven to 350F.

In a bowl, whisk together eggs, vinegar, coconut oil and honey. In separate bowl mix together coconut flour, almond flour, baking soda, cinnamon and salt. Unite the egg mixture with the flour mixture. Mix well. Add in the shredded carrots and sultana. Fill the muffin cups or cases. Bake for 30 minutes. Serve.

Servings: 12

Total Time: 45 minutes

Nutrition Facts

Serving size: 1/12 of a recipe (2,9 ounces).

Amount Per Serving	
Calories	231,15
Calories From Fat (42%)	96
	% Daily Value
Total Fat 11,06g	17%
Saturated Fat 8,43g	42%
Cholesterol 62mg	21%
Sodium 187,75mg	8%
Potassium 166,21mg	5%
Total Carbohydrates 30,99g	10%
Fiber 1,49g	6%
Sugar 16,8g	
Protein 4,15g	8%

Almond Inspiration Paleo Cookies

Ingredients

2 cups almond flour

2 eggs

4 Tbsp maple syrup

½ cup almonds, chopped

3 Tbsp coconut flour

1 cup cocoa powder

2 tsp vanilla extract

½ tsp baking soda

¼ tsp sea salt

Procedure

Preheat oven to 340F degrees.

In a bowl, whisk the eggs, coconut oil, maple syrup and vanilla extract. In a separate bowl, mix together the baking soda, almond flour, coconut flour, cocoa powder and salt. Unite the eggs mixture with the flour mixture. Pour dough in a greased baking pan. Sprinkle dough with chopped almond over top. Bake for 15-18 minutes. Let cool and cut into chunks. Serve.

Servings: 8

Total Time: 25 minutes

Nutrition Facts

Serving size: 1/8 of a recipe (5,7 ounces).

Amount Per Serving	
Calories	110,9
Calories From Fat (45%)	50
	% Daily Value
Total Fat 5,87g	9%
Saturated Fat 0,76g	4%
Cholesterol 46,5mg	16%
Sodium 781,6mg	33%
Potassium 109,56mg	3%
Total Carbohydrates 11,16g	4%
Fiber 1,12g	4%
Sugar 6,7g	
Protein 3,76g	8%

Classical Paleo Coconut Brownies

Ingredients

2 cup cocoa powder,

½ cup raw honey

1white sweet potato, grated

½ cup virgin olive oil

2 Tbsp coconut flour

2 eggs

2 tsp vanilla extract

½ Tbsp baking soda

1 Tbsp baking powder

¼ cup almonds, chopped

Procedure

Preheat oven to 360F degrees.

In a deep bowl, combine eggs, olive, grated potato, vanilla and honey. Stir until combined well. Add in baking soda and baking powder. Stir well. Finally, add in cocoa powder, coconut flour and chopped almonds. Stir well until combined well.

Pour the batter mixture in a greased (olive oil) baking pan. Bake for 30 minutes. When ready, leave on a wire rack to cool. You can melt down some cocoa powder in coconut milk and spread evenly over the top of brownies. Also, you can top brownies with your desired fruits. Cut into squares and serve.

Servings: 10

Total Time: 50 minutes

Nutrition Facts

Serving size: 1/10 of a recipe (2,1 ounces).

Amount Per Serving	
Calories	81,02
Calories From Fat (51%)	41,56
	% Daily Value
Total Fat 4,88g	8%
Saturated Fat 1,68g	8%
Cholesterol 37,2mg	12%
Sodium 354,26mg	15%
Potassium 292,75mg	8%
Total Carbohydrates 11,9g	4%
Fiber 5,5g	22%
Sugar 1,32g	
Protein 5,14g	10%

Halloween Paleo Pumpkin Pie

Ingredients	3 eggs
2 ½ cup pumpkin puree	1 ¼ Tbsp cinnamon
1 Paleo Pie Crust	1 Tbsp nutmeg
½ cup coconut milk	⅛ tsp sea salt
½ cup honey	

Procedure

Preheat oven to 360F degrees.

In a deep bowl, combine pumpkin puree and eggs. Pour in coconut milk, honey, nutmeg, cinnamon and salt. Stir it until combine well. Pour the batter in a pie crust. Bake for 45 minutes. When ready, let cool and put in refrigerator at least 3 hours before serving.

Servings: 8

Cooking Time: 55 minutes

Total Time: 3 hours and 55 minutes

Nutrition Facts

Serving size: 1/8 of a recipe (4,8 ounces).

Amount Per Serving	
Calories	168,68
Calories From Fat (32%)	53,76
	% Daily Value
Total Fat 6,23g	10%
Saturated Fat 3,89g	19%
Cholesterol 69,75mg	23%
Sodium 574,02mg	24%
Potassium 239,28mg	7%
Total Carbohydrates 27,45g	9%
Fiber 3,16g	13%
Sugar 20,27g	
Protein 3,79g	8%

Honey Apricot Paleo Muffins

Ingredients

1	cup apricots, diced
2	Tbsp coconut butter, melted
1	cup almond flour
3	eggs

2 Tbsp honey

1 ½ Tbsp lemon juice

½ tsp baking soda

¼ tsp sea salt

Procedure

Preheat oven to 340 degrees.

In a medium bowl, mix together flour, salt and baking soda. In a separate bowl, combine eggs, coconut butter, lemon juice and honey. Unit the both mixtures and fold in apricots.

Fill the muffin cups evenly. Bake for 30 minutes. Cool and serve.

Servings: 9

Total Time: 45 minutes

Nutrition Facts

Serving size: 1/9 of a recipe (2 ounces).

Amount Per Serving	
Calories	189,02
Calories From Fat (55%)	104,65
	% Daily Value
Total Fat 12,25g	19%
Saturated Fat 2,76g	14%
Cholesterol 68,78mg	23%
Sodium 703,61mg	29%
Potassium 305,82mg	9%
Total Carbohydrates 16,71g	6%
Fiber 2,78g	11%
Sugar 12,43g	
Protein 5,9g	12%

Orange Amaranth Paleo Cake

Ingredients   1 tsp nutmeg

¾ cup buckwheat flour   2 tsp sweetener (optional)

4 eggs   ½ cup cocoa powder

½ cup puffed amaranth   1 Tbsp cinnamon

4 Tbsp ghee   Pinch of salt

1 tsp orange essence

Procedure

Preheat oven to 300 ° F.

In a bowl, beat the eggs, ghee, salt, orange essence, spices while slowly adding the sifted flour. Add the amaranth and sweetener; continue mixing until you achieve the desired texture. Prepare a mold with wax or baking paper or grease with butter. Put the mixture into the mold. Cut up the cocoa powder and decorate the top.

Bake for 40 minutes. Once done, remove from oven and let cool on a rack. Serve and enjoy!

Servings: 8

Total Time: 55 minutes

Nutrition Facts

Serving size: 1/8 of a recipe (2,1 ounces).

Amount Per Serving	
Calories	89,82
Calories From Fat (36%)	32,14
	% Daily Value
Total Fat 3,66g	6%
Saturated Fat 1,43g	7%
Cholesterol 93mg	31%
Sodium 39,24mg	2%
Potassium 227,23mg	6%
Total Carbohydrates 12,35g	4%
Fiber 3,59g	14%
Sugar 1,24g	
Protein 5,78g	12%

Paleo Banana and Guava Biscuits

Ingredients	2 tsp cinnamon
1 ½ cup bananas	1 ½ tsp vanilla extract
½ cup guava, mashed	1 tsp baking soda
2 Tbsp coconut oil	¾ cup grated coconut
½ cup coconut flour	2 Tbsp dried plums or dried fruit (optional)

Procedure

Preheat oven to 360F. In a bowl, mix the bananas, mashed guava and vegetable shortening until it is fully combined.

In a bowl mix stir the flour, coconut, cinnamon, vanilla and baking soda. Add this mixture to the food processor to puree. Mix for 15 seconds.

At last, add the nuts and blend 1 minute more.

Make cookies with your hands. Place the cookies in a baking pan and bake 10-15 minutes. Turn biscuits on the other side and bake 15 minutes more. When ready, let cool on a wire rack. Serve.

Servings: 8

Total Time: 55 minutes

Nutrition Facts

Serving size: 1/8 of a recipe (2,8 ounces).

Amount Per Serving	
Calories	121,44
Calories From Fat (42%)	51,37
	% Daily Value
Total Fat 6,07g	9%
Saturated Fat 4,9g	25%
Cholesterol 0mg	0%
Sodium 171,97mg	7%
Potassium 193,84mg	6%
Total Carbohydrates 16,67g	6%
Fiber 1,76g	7%
Sugar 5,81g	
Protein 1,55g	3%

Paleo Orange and Hazelnuts Biscotti

Ingredients

2 cups almond flour

1/3 cup hazelnuts

½ cup orange juice

1 orange peel

2 Tbsp arrowroot tea

1 egg

6 dates

1 tsp ginger

½ tsp baking soda

3 Tbsp coconut oil

1 Tbsp cocoa powder

1 pinch of salt

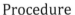

Procedure

Preheat oven to 360 ° C.

In a food processor, blend the dates together with hazelnuts until hazelnuts are chopped. Add the remaining ingredients and continue blending until mixed well. Form a ball with the batter. As it sticks a lot to your hands, just applied olive oil to mold it easier.

Put the dough on baking parchment paper, and extend it with your hands over the baking pan evenly. Bake for 20-25 minutes. When ready, remove tray from the oven and let batter cool. Once cooled, cut it. Put back in the oven and bake for about 10 minutes more. Cool and serve.

Servings: 14

Total Time: 50 minutes

Nutrition Facts

Serving size: 1/14 of a recipe (1,7 ounces).

Amount Per Serving	
Calories	184,55
Calories From Fat (71%)	131,64

	% Daily Value
Total Fat 15,61g	24%
Saturated Fat 3,6g	18%
Cholesterol 13,29mg	4%
Sodium 71,62mg	3%
Potassium 227,16mg	6%
Total Carbohydrates 9,08g	3%
Fiber 2,82g	11%
Sugar 4,64g	
Protein 5,13g	10%

Paleo Style Lime Cheesecake

Ingredients	For the filling
For the crust	¾ cup coconut oil, melted
2 cups almonds	1 cup lime juice
2 Tbsp coconut flakes	1 cup almond milk
¼ cup date paste	2 cups raw nuts
¼ tsp vanilla extract	¾ cup agave nectar
¼ tsp sea salt	1 tsp vanilla powder

Procedure

In a bowl, blend coconut flakes and almonds. Blend it well. Add in vanilla, salt and date paste. Blend until well combined. Place mixture into the pan and put in the fridge for 2 hours.

In a blender, mix the almond milk, agave nectar, lime juice, vanilla and row nuts about 30 seconds. Pour mixture into the pan with the cake crust. Freeze a cheesecake in the freezer about 3 hours. Before serving, decorate with lime zest and chopped almonds.

Servings: 14

Cooking Time: 15 minutes

Total Time: 5 hours

Nutrition Facts

Serving size: 1/14 of a recipe (3,7 ounces).

Amount Per Serving	
Calories	345,32
Calories From Fat (68%)	234,21
	% Daily Value
Total Fat 27,52g	42%
Saturated Fat 12,87g	64%
Cholesterol 1,39mg	<1%
Sodium 405,17mg	17%
Potassium 334,48mg	10%
Total Carbohydrates 22,08g	7%
Fiber 4,65g	19%
Sugar 13,56g	
Protein 7,2g	14%

Paleo Tempting Chocolate Cake

Ingredients

6 eggs

½ cup cocoa powder

¼ cup coconut milk

½ cup coconut flour

¾ cup coconut oil

½ cup honey

2 tsp vanilla

1 tsp baking soda

½ tsp white vinegar

½ tsp salt

Procedure

Preheat oven to 360 degrees F.

In a pot over low heat, mix the cocoa powder in coconut oil. Set aside to cool. In a deep bowl, blend eggs, vanilla, rice vinegar, honey and coconut milk. Add cooled cocoa mixture. In a separate bowl, mix the baking soda, coconut flour and salt. Unite the cocoa mixture with the egg mixture. Mix well.

Pour the batter blend in a greased baking pan. Bake for 30-35 minutes. When ready, leave to cool and serve.

Servings: 12

Total Time: 55 minutes

Nutrition Facts

Serving size: 1/12 of a recipe (2,2 ounces).

Amount Per Serving	
Calories	190,66
Calories From Fat (57%)	108,62
	% Daily Value
Total Fat 12,53g	19%
Saturated Fat 9,27g	46%
Cholesterol 93mg	31%
Sodium 239,59mg	10%
Potassium 130,6mg	4%
Total Carbohydrates 18,31g	6%
Fiber 1,59g	6%
Sugar 11,94g	
Protein 4,61g	9%

Strawberries Tart with Dried Cranberries

Ingredients	½ tsp	cinnamon
Tart - Base	1 tsp	vanilla extracts
1 cup coconut, desiccated	pinch	of salt
2 cup hazelnuts, roasted	Topping	
2 Tbsp cocoa	2 ¼ cup strawberries	
2 Tbsp coconut oil	fresh basil leaves	
1 cup raisins	1/3 cup cranberries, dried	

Procedure

In a pot boil the raisins. In a food processor put hazelnuts, coconut, cocoa, oil, cinnamon, vanilla and salt. Blend until crumbly. Add drain dates and continue to blend. Press mixture into a tart tin and put in the fridge for 1-2 hours. Slice the strawberries. Cover the tart with strawberries slices on top and sprinkle the dried cranberries over. Decorate with fresh basil leaves. Keep refrigerated.

Servings: 12

Cooking Time: 10 minutes

Total Time: 3 hours and 10 minutes

Nutrition Facts

Serving size: 1/12 of a recipe (3,1 ounces).

Amount Per Serving		% Daily Value
Calories		260,75
Calories From Fat (50%)		129,89
Total Fat 15,43g		24%
Saturated Fat 4,78g		24%
Cholesterol 0mg		0%
Sodium 3,97mg		<1%
Potassium 318,5mg		9%
Total Carbohydrates 31,19g		10%
Fiber 4,67g		19%
Sugar 10,82g		
Protein 3,52g		7%

Bonus – 7 days Body cleanse & Detox

If you feel that you are constantly tired, sleepy and that you do not have enough energy, it is a time for an awesome body cleanse! Green leaves used in green smoothies are full of indissoluble fibers that are essential to eliminate the toxins and waste accumulated in the body. It will help your digestive system, make you feel fresh and verve, improve mental clarity and prevent many diseases. Seriously, I remember the first time I did 7 days of this and boy did I feel good. Keep in mind most of your weight loss will be water weight which you will put back on once you start eating solids but this is all about detox and feeling the fresh energy. This will maximise your productivity as you will be very energised!

Doing a juice cleanse has been said to help unleash the natural healing power of your body by getting rid of all those yucky built up toxins. Juicing floods your system with powerful nutrients and antioxidants. It may be the first step towards a long-lasting lifestyle change, or jumpstarting a weight-loss regimen by helping to retrain your taste buds as well as psychological connection to food. Use colorful juice cleanses packed with so much delicious goodness and you'll never believe something so healthy can be so satisfying.

CHAPTER 9

BONUS SECTION: KEEPING A WELL-STOCKED PANTRY

Nothing makes cooking more frustrating than not having all of the ingredients needed to make something truly delicious. This bonus section will help you keep your pantry well-stocked and ready for whatever inspiration comes your way!

The Gluten-Free (GF) Pantry

Gluten is a protein—technically a mix of proteins—found in some cereal grains. People with celiac disease and gluten allergies cannot tolerate gluten and must avoid it at all costs. For the general population, a growing body of research suggests eliminating gluten will help prevent obesity, diabetes, cardiovascular problems, and digestive disorders like "leaky gut syndrome."

There's also persuasive evidence of a connection between gluten allergies and the onset of Alzheimer's and other dementia. (This has been dubbed "grain brain.")

When living gluten-free is a health imperative rather than simply a dietary choice, it's particularly important to read labels. Gluten can lurk in the most unlikely places (in the malt vinegar you've just sprinkled on your fish and chips, for instance) and words like bulgur, spelt, triticale, and malt can all spell trouble.

WHAT TO STOCK:
- Seeds
- Nuts, nut butters, and nut oils
- Peanuts and peanut butters
- Dried beans and lentils
- Dried fruit
- Larabars—advertised as the "original fruit and nut bar," these treats are contain nothing but fruit, nuts, and spices. (Note: these snacks should not be eaten by those on a weight-loss diet or those with blood sugar issues as they are rank very high on the glycemic index.)
- Blue Diamond Nut thins
- Jerky
- Potato Chips
- Corn tortillas
- Oatmeal certified GF
- Rice Chex or other rice-based cold cereal (Glutino has four different options of cold cereal)
- If your local supermarket/health food store does not carry your favorite brand of GF cereal, try one of the mail order sources like Arrowhead Mills or Bob's Red Mill Natural Foods.

- Rice, brown rice, black rice, wild rice
- Quinoa, millet, amaranth
- Cornmeal

For Baking:
- Almond flour
- Coconut flour
- Arrowroot powder
- Cornstarch
- Tapioca starch
- Gluten-free baking mixes
- There are now a variety of excellent gluten-free baking mixes available, like the ones sold by Bob's Red Mill and Pamela's.
- Honey, Maple Syrup, Blue Agave Syrup

Condiments:
- All herbs, dried and fresh.
- Spices and spice blends (curry powder, chili powder) that do not include additives like sugar or salt.
- Dried seaweed sheets and flakes
- GF soy sauce
- Bragg's Liquid aminos
- Coconut aminos (to substitute for soy sauce, which is made from a legume). If you can't find them in your local supermarket, health or whole foods store, they are readily available online.
- Distilled hot pepper sauces (like Tabasco)
- Mustard, ketchup, mayonnaise, relish

In the Fridge:
- Dairy products, including milk, yogurt, sour cream, and cheese
- Almond Milk
- Soy milk
- Coconut milk
- Eggs
- Unprocessed meat (no hotdogs and especially no corn dogs!)
- Frozen vegetables without sauce
- Frozen fruit without added sugar or sauce
- Gluten-free pie crust

BONUS TOOL FOR GLUTEN-FREE DIETERS: A RICE COOKER

A kitchen-sized version of the giant rice pots found in Asian restaurants, this appliance allows a cook to dump in the rice, water, seasonings and other ingredients, set the timer and walk away. The rice comes out perfect every time, with no burnt crust or soupiness.

The Paleo Pantry

The Paleo diet (also dubbed the "Caveman Diet") is built around the simple concept that eating only the foods available to our ancient hunter/gatherer ancestors is the best way to avoid modern health problems like obesity, Type II diabetes, cardiovascular disease, and cancer.

The Paleo diet is an omnivorous eating plan that includes animal protein, fish, fruits, most vegetables (potatoes are forbidden), seeds, nuts, and vegetable-based fats.

The Paleo diet does NOT include dairy, sugar, grains, legumes, alcohol, or processed foods of any kind except those that have been dehydrated, like raisins and other dried fruit.

Some food lists are stricter than others and there's some disagreement over the inclusion or exclusion of honey, maple syrup, chocolate, coffee, vinegar, and wine. Tailor your diet to your needs, and be realistic. If you want a little dark chocolate or a glass or red wine occasionally, it's not going to throw your eating plan into complete disarray. "Moderation in all things" should be the goal.

WHAT TO STOCK:
- Seeds
- Nuts, nut butters, and nut oils
- Remember, peanuts are not nuts, they're legumes; so no peanuts, peanut butter or peanut oil.
- Olive oil
- Coconut oil
- Dried fruit
- Larabars—advertised as the "original fruit and nut bar," these treats are not just Paleo, they're also gluten-free containing fruit, nuts, and spices. (Note: these snacks should not be eaten by those on a weight-loss diet or those with blood sugar issues as they are rank very high on the glycemic index.)
- Jerky, preferably made without sugar.

Condiments:
- All herbs, dried and fresh.
- Spices and spice blends (curry powder, chili powder) that do not include additives like sugar or salt.
- Dried seaweed sheets and flakes
- Distilled pepper sauces like Tabasco
- Coconut aminos (to substitute for soy sauce, which is made from a legume). If you can't find them in your local supermarket, health or whole foods store, they are readily available online.
- Mustard without additives or thickeners. (You can make your own by mixing mustard or wasabi powder with water.)

- Commercial mayonnaise and ketchup are off the Paleo table. You can make mayonnaise from egg yolks and oil, and ketchup created from scratch.

For Baking:
- Almond flour
- Coconut flour
- Arrowroot powder
- Tapioca starch

In the Fridge:
- Coconut Milk
- Almond Milk
- Eggs
- Frozen vegetables without sauce
- Frozen fruit without added sugar or sauce
- Unprocessed meat (no hotdogs and especially no corn dogs!)
- Beef, pork, lamb, and poultry make up the bulk of animal protein consumed today but the options available in grocery stores already goes far beyond those four meat selections. Ethnic markets often have goat in stock. Rabbit is readily available in the freezer section of most large supermarkets, and in large cities, it's easy to find ground buffalo and ostrich (a red meat) as well. Especially during the winter holidays, many stores allow patrons to special order "exotic" turkey alternates like goose, pheasant, and quail.
- All these meats—and even more exotic victuals like alligator and rattlesnake—are available by mail order.

BONUS TOOL FOR PALEO DIETERS: A DEHYDRATOR

Raw foodists have perfected the art of making crackers and "breads" from seeds with a hydrator. Making meat and fish jerky in a dehydrator is an easy and more energy-efficient process than making it an oven.

Weight-Loss Pantry

Being overweight stresses out your body and contributes to increased risk of heart attack, stroke, diabetes, and cancer. If extra weight is coupled with other risk factors, like smoking or excess alcohol consumption, there's a multiplier effect.

There are a number of effective weight-loss eating plans—from low-carb to high-fiber to low fat—but the outcome of any diet is a matter of simple math. You have to expend more calories than you consume. The best way to accomplish your weight-loss goals is to focus on whole foods, nutrition-dense fruits and vegetables, whole grains, healthy dairy, and quality protein. The more processed a food is, the more chemicals it contains, the less likely it is to be nutritious and satisfying. (It's easy to eat a whole bag of potato chips without putting a dent in your appetite but not as easy to eat a bag of fiber-rich carrots.)

No matter which diet plan you choose to attain your weight loss, getting back to basics and eating "clean" is a good place to start.

When you first embark on a weight-loss regimen, it's tempting to stock up on diet this and low-fat that. But if you're filling your pantry with non-fat cookies and diet soda, you're missing the point. It's also tempting to rely on pre-packed diet meals, either the frozen kind or the dehydrated ones that are delivered monthly to your door. Some of these packaged foods are so filled with preservatives that their sell-by date is not for another decade. Stick with real food.

WHAT TO STOCK:
- Seeds
- Nuts, nut butters, and nut oils
- Peanuts and peanut butters
- Seeds and nuts are good for dieters. A handful of nuts (an ounce or so) makes a satisfying snack thanks to the fat. But practice portion control; it's easy to eat a lot of seeds or nuts in a single sitting.
- Dried popcorn (not the microwave kind)
- Dried beans and lentils
- Dried fruit
- Jerky
- Corn tortillas
- Oatmeal
- Brown rice, wild rice, quinoa, millet, amaranth
- Don't use white rice, it ranks 64 on the glycemic index (GI), and even a small portion can spike blood sugar.
- Whole Wheat flour
- Buckwheat flour
- Honey, Maple Syrup, Blue Agave Syrup
- There are a wide variety of artificial sweeteners on the marketplace. It's counter-intuitive, but some research suggests that these substances can trigger everything from bloating and belly fat production to the onset of Type 2 diabetes. It's better to avoid them altogether and use healthier alternatives. If you must use an artificial sweetener, make it a natural one, like Stevia.
- Coconut oil
- Canola oil
- Olive oil
- Sesame oil
- Vinegar—any kind except flavored vinegars with added sugar. Balsamic vinegar is high in sugar, so use it in moderation.
- Stay away from all commercial salad dressings. They are loaded with salt and sugar, often shockingly so. They also tend to have a lot of preservatives added for long shelf-life. Make your own salad dressing.

Condiments:
- All herbs, dried and fresh
- Spices and spice blends (curry powder, chili powder) that do not include additives like sugar or salt
- Dried seaweed sheets and flakes
- Low-sodium soy sauce
- Distilled hot pepper sauces (like Tabasco)
- Mustard
- Most dieters avoid mayonnaise but it's really ketchup that's the worst condiment culprit. Loaded with sugar, salt, added thickeners and preservatives, putting ketchup on your food is like pouring thick syrup over it. Try one of the organic brands at the health food store if you must have ketchup.

In the Fridge:
- Milk, cheese, Greek yogurt
- When it comes to dairy products, "low fat and non-fat" aren't necessarily the best choices for a weight-loss diet. In one oft-quoted study conducted at the University of Tennessee, researchers found that subjects who were fed a diet rich in whole milk lost more belly fat than those given low-fat or no-fat dairy. And while the findings are controversial, other research suggests that the added fat in whole milk actually boosts fat-burning. If you want a glass of whole milk, go ahead, just don't blend it into a milkshake if you want to lose weight.
- Eggs
- Unprocessed meat—stay away from processed meats like bologna, lunch meats, and hot dogs. Bacon can be included in a low-carb regimen, but if possible, choose an uncured, sugar-free, nitrate-free brand. There are a number of mail-order sources for these brands if they are not available in your local area.
- Frozen vegetables without sauce
- Frozen fruit without added sugar or sauce
- Frozen fish without breading

BONUS TOOL FOR GLUTEN-FREE DIETERS: A SLOW COOKER

Slow cookers are larger than crockpots and allow a cook more flexibility. Either appliance is useful for creating stews, soups, spaghetti sauce, and chilis, but the slow-cooker allows for bigger batches at a time, which is a boon for the busy cook. Making food ahead and freezing individual portions means that there's always something good to eat in the length of time it takes to microwave the meal.